# Wartime Nurse

*By the same author*

Front Line City – Cologne
Yorkshire at War
York Blitz
Operation Millennium: Bomber Harris's
 Raid on Cologne, May 1942
Women Who Went to War: 1938–46
Forces Sweethearts: Service Romances in World War II
Heroines of World War II
Showbiz Goes to War
Front-line Nurse
Combat Nurse

# WARTIME NURSE

*One Hundred Years from the Crimea
to Korea 1854–1954*

ERIC TAYLOR

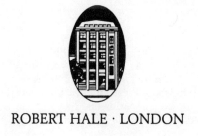

ROBERT HALE · LONDON

© Eric Taylor 2001
First published in Great Britain 2001

ISBN 0 7090 6777 1

Robert Hale Limited
Clerkenwell House
Clerkenwell Green
London EC1R 0HT

2 4 6 8 10 9 7 5 3 1

*A catalogue record for this book is available from the British Library*

Typeset in Revival by
Derek Doyle & Associates, Liverpool.
Printed in Great Britain by
St Edmundsbury Press, Bury St Edmunds, Suffolk
and bound by
Woolnough Bookbinding Limited, Irthlingborough

# Contents

# Acknowledgements

In writing this book I have again been fortunate in having invaluable help from headquarters staff of the nursing services and the Army Medical Museum.

It is with warm gratitude that I also acknowledge my debt to the staff of the Public Record Office, the Imperial War Museum Department of Documents, the National Newspaper Library at Colindale, the BBC Film Archives and the United States National Archives. Without their generous and ready help this book would not have been so comprehensive.

My sincere thanks are due to so many former nurses, military personnel and their relatives, too numerous to mention by name here but I trust they will accept this brief expression of my gratitude along with the thanks I have already expressed personally to them all. They were able to supply me with memoirs of service in South Africa, both world wars and Korea. I am particularly grateful for help from former Nursing Sister Jill Hall, now McNair, David Oates, Wyndham Davidson, F. Ellison, and Ashley Cunningham-Boothe, whose book, *British Forces in the Korean War* compiled with Peter Farrar has been a great help to me. It was in this book that I was also to read accounts of life aboard the hospital ship, HMHS *Maine* written by former Matron Ruth Stone, QARNNS. They were most informative. Once again I appreciated help from Charles Whiting who made available to me his research for his book *Battleground Korea*.

I am indebted also to Marie Stride for her help and access to her comprehensive book *Celebrating Salisbury Nurses*. I owe special thanks too for the help I received from Alec Adamson and his detailed and most interesting memoirs of service in Military Hospitals in England, the Sudan and the Western Desert from 1939 until the cessation of hostilities.

I would rather belatedly like to pay tribute to two people who unknowingly at the time told me so much about nursing in World War

6

One; they are my mother, then Nurse Edith Stout, and my father, Sergeant Wilfred Taylor, serving in France with the Royal Army Medical Corps, but I pay tribute to them here nevertheless.

As with my other two books on wartime nurses – *Front-line Nurse* and *Combat Nurse* – I owe an immense debt to my wife Sheila who was so often able to help with the interviewing of former nurses and with the research.

To everyone I express my sincere thanks. The responsibility for any shortcomings or errors is, of course, my own.

# Glossary

| | |
|---|---|
| ADMS | Assistant Director of Medical Services |
| ADS | Advance Dressing Station |
| ATS | Auxiliary Territorial Service |
| CAEC | Casualty Air Evacuation Centre |
| CCS | Casualty Clearing Station |
| CO | Commanding Officer |
| DADMS | Deputy Assistant Director of Medical Services |
| DSO | Distinguished Service Order |
| DZ | Dropping Zone |
| FANY | First Aid Nursing Yeomanry |
| FAP | First Aid Post |
| FDS | Field Dressing Station |
| FSU | Field Surgical Unit |
| GOC | General Officer Commanding |
| HQ | Headquarters |
| LCI | Landing Craft Infantry |
| LCT | Landing Craft Tank |
| MC | Military Cross |
| MO | Medical Officer |
| NCO | Non-Commissioned Officer |
| OC | Officer Commanding |
| OR | Other Rank |
| OTT | Operating Theatre Technician |
| POW | Prisoner of War |
| QAIMNS | Queen Alexandra's Imperial Military Nursing Service |
| QARANC | Queen Alexandra's Royal Army Nursing Corps |
| QARNNS | Queen Alexandra's Royal Naval Nursing Service |
| QM | Quartermaster |
| RAP | Regimental Aid Post |
| RMO | Regimental Medical Officer |

8

| | |
|---|---|
| SMO | Senior Medical Officer |
| TA | Territorial Army |
| TCV | Troop-carrying vehicle |
| UN | United Nations |
| VAD | Voluntary Aid Detachments |
| WAAF | Women's Auxiliary Air Force |
| WRNS | Women's Royal Navy Service |
| WTS | Women's Transport Service |

# Illustrations

Margaret Nesbit RRC (Retd) and Major Diana Wilson (Retd)
50   Jill McNair outside the United Nations Command Advance HQ,
     Camp Boniface, September 1990

## Illustration Credits

Lea Hurst Collection, Derbyshire: 1. Bryn Purdy: 2. QARANC
Museum: 3, 10. QARNNS Archives: 4. Imperial War Museum,
London: 5, 6, 8, 32, 35. *Yorkshire Post*: 7. Army Medical Services
Museum: 9, 13, 15, 17. Family of Lilly Grace Petter: 11. Louise
Jefferson: 12. George Scott Collection: 18. Eleanor Pickering: 19, 20,
28. Violet Leather and Salisbury Nurses League: 21. Helen Long: 22.
Marie Floyd-Norris: 23, 24. Joan Ottaway: 25. Gladys Spencer
Crichton: 26. Edna Viner: 27. Malta Museum of World War Two: 29.
RAF Museum: 30, 31, 33. US Army Signal Corps: 34. Derek Ball: 36,
37. Australian War Memorial: 38, 41. Beatrice Hownam: 40. Jill
McNair: 42, 43, 47, 48, 49, 50. Alec Adamson: 44. David Oates: 45.

All other photographs are from the author's collection

# 1 Send Them Some Nurses!

'It will be difficult to find women equal to the task after all the horrors of the situation are known.'[1]

Sidney Herbert, Secretary of State for War, 1854

It was a sign of the times. Twenty-two years of peace after the Napoleonic wars and provocative newspaper reports against the 'Russian monster' had brought Victorian Britain to a strange condition of actually welcoming war. They clamoured for it. Or so said the newspapers, with banner headlines such as 'Ripe and Ready for the Fray', and cartoons showing a maiden in distress – 'Poor little Turkey' – with 'Britannia' coming to her aid. For a year the country had expected war. Now the day had come. Troops were on the march.

Crowds lined the streets all over London. With patriotic fervour they cheered their soldiers off to war. From St George's Barracks, Trafalgar Square, the Coldstream Guards swung proudly out of the gates, buttons sparkling, behind the regimental band playing a jaunty march-time arrangement of 'The Girl I Left Behind Me'. It was an appropriate tune, some might have said, on that bitterly cold 14 February 1854. The more perceptive ones in the crowd, though, knew this was not a day for celebrating with Valentine cards. Few of those young guardsmen would ever return to the girls they left behind.

Listening to the sound of marching bands through the palace windows, 35-year-old Queen Victoria was not at all happy to hear the soldiers of the Queen marching forth to war. Despite the emotions roused by the military music she was perturbed and wrote that day to her uncle: 'My heart is not in this unsatisfactory war.'[2]

The destination of those troops was a remote promontory on the Black Sea, the Crimea, two thousand miles from London. Their ultimate invasion beach had the foreboding name, Kalamita Bay.

What no one realized was that soon, British nurses would also be there. In the oppressive heat of summer and the long sub-zero months of winter, they would experience officially for the first time military service in a combat zone.

From barracks all over the southern counties now the pitifully small British army converged towards the embarkation ports, cheered all the way by enthusiastic crowds – crowds that had previously looked on soldiers as little better than drunken thugs and layabouts who had joined the army because they could not get a better job. Times now were different.

The excitement continued as each day went by. Deafening cheers greeted the line of small drummer boys leading the battalion of the Scottish Fusiliers out of their barracks, swinging their arms impressively high with all the parade-ground swank their sergeant-major had drilled into them.

As the column reached the corner, a small boy standing on the pavement with his dog came to attention and saluted gravely. Equally grave in his office that morning was the prime minister, Lord Aberdeen, who deplored the way Britain was being driven into war by a kind of public hysteria. He dreaded the consequence of it all.

Vehemently too he resented the way one ambitious politician in particular was pushing the country into the bloody conflict it was bound to be. It was Lord Palmerston, motivated, thought Aberdeen, into espousing an aggressive war attitude to improve his own popularity and political prospects. Like many politicians before and after him, he realized how much pursuing a bellicose line could dramatically enhance his own popularity with the voting public.

Nothing seemed to dampen the war hysteria that gripped the capital. The cheering crowds somehow assumed they were sending off their men to a victory like that of Waterloo, but they did not know how scandalously those soldiers had been prepared for the conflict; how deficient the army was in armament and training. Its artillery comprised a mere forty field-pieces that inspectors had already described as 'defective' and some infantry units still had old muskets from the Napoleonic wars. And it was under the command of Lord Raglan, a 66-year-old general, who had not seen active service for forty years.

Treasury penny-pinching, popular with tax-paying voters, meant soldiers being sent to fight a war with inadequate weaponry, little experience in large-scale military exercises, and insufficient medical and nursing care. There were no professional nurses, no trained stretcher-bearers, no means of transporting casualties from battlefield to casualty stations or field hospitals, and no adequate provision of medical supplies and hospital food. The army went to war with the same old tradition of living off the country in which it was fighting. A civilian commissariat officer went with the regiment and was responsible for providing food, liquor and forage for horses. For such a man forms and signatures were of paramount importance. Items for medical care came far down his list of army requisitions.

As for the Royal Navy, which the British public always believed to be superior to all others, in 1854 it was mostly laid up in harbour, dismantled aloft and disarmed below, in a limbo of its transition from sail to steam.

Worst of all, though, were the soldiers themselves. They were hardly physically fit enough to fight, as nurses would soon discover. They might have impressed the cheering crowds with their marching but they were far from being tough enough to fight a campaign under the winter conditions of the Crimea.

For years they had lived in squalid insanitary barracks on a diet little better than that of a pauper. As no army cooks were provided men took cookhouse duty in turns, with results not in the best practice of hygiene in surroundings frequently pestilential. Not surprisingly, men had little resistance to the diseases they would shortly meet. In fact, so unhealthy were these soldiers that their mortality rate in peace time was statistically twice that of civilians of the same age groups.

The public could be forgiven for not knowing how ill-prepared was Britain's military machine, but Palmerston, as a cabinet minister, and the national newspapers urging the country to war and criticizing the prime minister's attitude of appeasement, should have known better. Nevertheless, they pursued a course foredooming twenty-five thousand of their countrymen to an unnecessary and painful death, with inadequate medical and nursing care.

At that time, each regiment was supposed to have its own medical officer who belonged to the civil department of the army and held no commissioned rank. In peace time his main task was to sort out the malingerers and send them back to duty. Those he could not treat were sent to a regimental hospital where they were cared for by a hospital doctor and male ward orderlies seconded for duty from the regiment, usually because they were unfit for any other duty. These orderlies had no formal training in nursing, but over the years some of them had picked up a certain amount of medical knowledge from being on the job.

In military hospitals the army employed no trained cooks. As with the regiments, men took turns to be duty cook. As nurses in the

Crimea were soon to find out, no one ever thought of preparing nourishing meals for the very sick or wounded.

In 1854 there were officially no women nurses in military hospitals. Indeed, the medical profession was a man's world. It was
unthinkable that a woman from a good home should become a nurse.
Even women working in civil hospitals were looked upon as sluts who
did the dirty tasks and were given an occasional swig of beer for any
particularly unpleasant duty. In military hospitals early in the nineteenth century though, there were some women, because as well as
the traditional camp followers there were also wives who followed
the troops at home and overseas. For a short time after the
Napoleonic wars, a few women, poorly paid soldiers' wives, worked
in some military hospitals, carrying out domestic duties, but gradually
their number decreased until none remained by the end of the 1840s.
Thus, as the troops marched out to their embarkation ports in the
winter of 1854, the army medical system was an understaffed male
preserve with a strong antipathy towards the idea of employing
women as nurses.

In defence of that male attitude to women nurses we should bear
in mind that in peace time a quarter of all admissions to military
hospitals were for venereal disease. Male nurses were considered to
be more suitable for these patients. The attitude of army doctors was
that the bedside of a dying soldier was not the place for a respectable
young woman to be. 'The conviction was for a soldier to die hard,'
wrote Major General John Beith.[3]

However, the day that women nurses would transform those
hospitals was not far off.

On 23 February 1854, the first draft of troops in their picturesque
but unserviceable uniforms went aboard the three liners converted as
troopships, the *Ripon*, *Orinoco* and *Manilla*. They sailed out together
into a stormy Solent, bound for a war whose underlying causes, and
even location, few soldiers on board were aware of. Vaguely they
heard that Britain was in alliance with France against the tyranny of
Russia.

The more informed of the British public knew that the Turkish (or
Ottoman) Empire, which for so long had held the Balkan peninsula
together, had grown so weak, corrupt and militarily ineffective that
France and Britain began to fear that Russia would move into the area,
seize Constantinople and thereby threaten Britain's route to India.

In France, the self-appointed dictator, Louis Napoleon III, saw an
opportunity for self-aggrandisement by joining Britain in an alliance
against Russia. It was at his prompting that French and British fleets

were sent to close the Black Sea to Russian naval operations. He too feared Russia would dominate the Mediterranean if she seized Constantinople.

From then on, rivalry and fear became motives that impelled nations to war. On 28 March 1854 Britain and France declared war on Russia – a war that many far-sighted politicians predicted would be hard to wage and all but impossible to bring to a successful conclusion. And it was in such conditions that the need for good nursing care became so tragically obvious. Fortunately Victorian women were already being inspired to become war nurses. War fever was affecting everyone.

Sadly, from the beginning of the campaign it seemed that everything was doomed to failure. Britain's army then numbered 60,000 men – less than a sixth of the size of the Russian army. It was destined by the criminal mismanagement and incompetence of its senior commanders to endure months of almost indescribable torment and to suffer appalling casualties.

A force of two thousand British soldiers landing at Constantinople was almost immediately despatched three hundred miles up the Black Sea to Varna. There Lord Raglan had established his headquarters, in readiness for the first clash with the Russian army at Alma.

In the almost insufferable heat of Varna the British and French gathered for their first engagement with the Russian army. It was then that men began to fall out of the march clutching their bellies in great pain and vomiting. The tougher ones carried on, but suffering terrible thirst and feeling completely exhausted. The onset was so rapid it frightened others. One day a man was alive and marching and the next dead. Those who did get back to base for primitive medical care looked like the dead already, with their skin cold and blue-tinged, dry and shrunken. With faces pinched they collapsed close to the lavatory trenches as diarrhoea gripped them. Hundreds of them! Clearly these were not men malingering but men wracked with pain. So many died where they lay. Some dropped dead in their tracks.

Even to the least experienced of those doctors the symptoms were classic enough for diagnosis – just as the book said – 'patient cyanosed, incontinent and semi-conscious'.

Cholera!

The news shocked everyone, and like the disease itself spread with terrifying swiftness from one regiment to another. It attacked the Light Division, the 3rd Division, and some of the cavalry regiments. No one seemed to know how best to treat these men. Within days a full-scale epidemic was rampaging through the ranks. Its mortality was terrifying. In hospitals, doctors seemed helpless. No one had any experience of nursing these patients. All kinds of remedies and treatments were tried. Some doctors believed the disease came from breathing impure air, so they actually ordered men to smoke in the hospital wards to help prevent the spread of the disease! Others experimented with chloroform; they dosed patients with brandy and ice, and rubbed their cramped joints and stomach with turpentine and mustard. Most treatments were futile.

Despite their ranks being ravaged by disease, the British and French armies marched on for their first battle against the Russians at the Alma. In the blazing September sun they trudged for miles across dry, treeless plains without a drop of water to be got on the way. Advancing on a front four miles wide, with scarlet uniforms and glittering brasses, they must have made a picturesque though tragic spectacle.

The Russian army, Dragoons and Cossacks waited for them on the other side of the River Alma. By this time, 20 September 1854, the French and British soldiers were exhausted. The battle began with an artillery bombardment and both the British and French made good ground but suddenly got the order to retire. Troops fell back, angry and bewildered. Eventually out of the confusion came further orders to advance and the Russians, equally bewildered, were thoroughly defeated.

The British and French were then in a position to turn victory into a rout. But the opportunity to pursue the defeated Russians was not taken. Historians have since argued that if the attack had been pushed home, the city of Sebastapol might well have been taken. Instead the war was to drag on for two years and at a cost of nearly 300,000 casualties.

On the other hand, others believe the two armies did exceedingly well to be victorious in the first battle of the Alma with their divisions ravaged by cholera. Ironically, too, wounded men who went back to base hospitals increased their chances of getting the dreaded cholera.

No one at base knew what to do with cholera casualties.

But there were nurses in Britain with experience of caring for cholera patients. In the summer of 1854 an epidemic of cholera had broken out in London, the hospitals were overcrowded and many nurses died. Others, fearing infection, simply ran away.

In the midst of that outbreak in London, a tall, short-haired woman with a willowy figure reported to the Senior Medical Officer of the Middlesex Hospital and volunteered to superintend the nursing of cholera patients from the epidemic. For days afterwards she was rarely off her feet receiving panic-stricken women, many of them crazed with drink and fear. Soon they learnt to be quiet and do as they were told by this strange woman with a gentle manner but with a will, described by her colleague, Mrs Gaskell, as 'of cold, hard steel'.

Her name was Florence Nightingale.

Born in Florence in the summer of 1820, a year after Queen Victoria, she had studied hospital administration and management in Germany, gained further experience by working in a hospital and orphanage there and studied sanitation and hygiene. Still seeking further experience she spent a short time in Paris at the hospital of the Sisters of Mercy. She returned home to be in charge of a small hospital for 'gentlewomen' in Harley Street, London, and it was a year later when she offered her services to the Middlesex Hospital.

Florence Nightingale epitomized the calibre of nurses needed then by the soldiers in the Crimea. Unfortunately no one had thought women nurses had a place in military hospitals in 1854. But the nursing situation in hospitals there was critical. In those first three months of June, July and August, 20 per cent of the entire Crimean Expeditionary Force was hospitalized. Nearly a thousand of those soldiers died before a shot was fired.

Daily the problem of caring for casualties got worse. In addition to all those cholera patients in the barrack hospital at Scutari, there came wounded men from renewed battles around Sebastapol. They were brought in makeshift hospital ships, where the wounded lay bleeding alongside groaning cholera cases.

One ship, the *Kangaroo*, mentioned in a report to *The Times*, had 1,500 casualties crammed together on the floor below decks in a space planned for 250. The report told how, during a rough sea crossing, most of the wounded were seasick and too weak to step over bodies to go to the few lavatories, so they defecated and urinated where they lay, and as the ship rolled, so men rolled together into one huge filthy heap. Men with legs and arms amputated, were flung about screaming in agony.

When those makeshift hospital ships reached the port at Scutari there was no relief for the casualties on board. As there were no beds for them in the hospital, patients were laid on the floor, still in the blood-soaked blankets and uniform in which they had travelled from the battlefield. Neither food nor drink was immediately available because no kitchen was working, and there were not even cups or mugs from which drinks could be given. There was no furniture nor even an operating table.

For the first time in the history of their wars, relatives of the soldiers and the general public were able to keep up with the news from the front. It was a new era, the time of railways and steamships and, more important still, the time of the newly invented electric telegraph. No longer were people back home having to rely solely on out-of-date communiqués from general officers who conveniently omitted from their reports the unpleasant aspects of war such as casualties and terrible living conditions. Now also soldiers were better educated, and they wrote letters home describing the sort of life they were living. But for the graphic details then, official war correspondents were on the spot.

They portrayed vividly the horror of it all. They penetrated everywhere in the combat zone; questioned commanders and private soldiers; visited the wounded and sent disturbing reports back to their editors. Now the public at home who had cheered their menfolk off to war could see what the conflict really meant for them. They saw a frightened picture and, worse still, a mishandled war. Especially notable were reports by the Irish journalist, William Russell of *The Times*, on 9 and 12 October 1854.

He denounced in the most explicit words the shameful lack of arrangements for the nursing of the sick and wounded. 'It is with feelings of surprise and anger that the public will learn that insufficient preparations have been made for the care of the wounded. Not only are there not enough surgeons, not only are there not enough bandages, *but there are no nurses.*'

He spared no one's feelings in depicting scenes of horror. 'Soldiers bleeding to death are left to die untended!' He argued that British casualties were far greater than they need have been. In another report he wrote:

> There is no preparation for the commonest of surgical operations! Not only are the men kept, in some cases, for a week without the hand of a medical man coming near their wounds, not only are they left to expire in agony, unheeded and shaken off, though clutching desperately at the surgeon whenever he makes his rounds through the fetid ship, but now when they are placed in a spacious building, at Scutari, where we were led to believe that everything was ready which could ease their pain and facilitate their recovery, it is found that the commonest appliances of a workhouse sick-ward are wanting.[4]

> The worn out pensioners who were brought out as an Ambulance Corps are totally useless, and not only are surgeons not to be had,

but there are no dressers or nurses to carry out the surgeons' instructions.

The news burst upon the British public like a thunderclap and left them seething with rage especially when they read that the French army had Sisters of Charity to look after their soldiers – 'devoted women who were excellent nurses'. Not surprisingly a forceful letter appeared in the next edition of *The Times*, asking, 'Why don't the British have Sisters of Charity?'

The attitude immediately taken by women at home was, certainly if French women could withstand the hardships of life nursing in the Crimea then so too could English women. Once roused, the British public started to act. A fund was set up to provide medical necessities and comfort for sick and wounded soldiers.

Hastily the army denied there was anything amiss. False reports were fabricated and despatched to London. But Sidney Herbert, secretary at war, was not reassured by army accounts that looked more like a cover-up than a genuine assessment. He wrote immediately to the Middlesex Hospital to ask whether Miss Nightingale would take a party of nurses to Scutari and be in charge of their organization in the hospital there at government expense and with official support.

Herbert had met Florence Nightingale seven years earlier in Rome and both he and his wife had become firm friends, kindred spirits with genuine feelings for the welfare of the poor and for soldiers in particular. He had been particularly impressed by her efficiency as superintendent of the hospital for the care of sick gentlewomen.

Furthermore he immediately authorized the British ambassador at Constantinople to buy all that was required by the hospitals at Scutari.

As it happened, Florence Nightingale was already a step ahead of him. She had been picking nurses of her own accord to go with her to the Crimea. That selection had not been easy. Most of the women who applied to go to the Crimea as nurses were motivated solely by the pay and some of them were from very rough backgrounds. She feared the promiscuity shown by women camp followers in previous wars and so made it known to all applicants that any misconduct with the troops would result in instant dismissal. On the other hand, the nurses who were eventually chosen were not, as is often represented, fine ladies of breeding. Although born into the upper classes herself she had no time for 'fine ladies' whose idea of nursing amounted to nothing more than stroking a soldier's brow and straightening his pillow. Nor was she keen on the sisters of religious orders. She once caustically described them as: 'fit more for heaven than a hospital. They flit about like angels without hands among the patients and soothe their souls while they leave their bodies dirty and neglected.'

Those finally selected were a workaday group, some without Miss Nightingale's spirit of devotion; but in the Scutari hospital they were moulded into an efficient staff by their superintendent's strict discipline.

Sidney Herbert had known he was asking a lot of Florence Nightingale, for there were not many trained nurses of the right calibre available. He too was fully aware that women who nursed soldiers sometimes had a reputation for offering services more sexual than therapeutic. In his letter to Miss Nightingale he had written: 'The selection of the rank and file nurses will be very difficult; no one knows it better than yourself.'

Prophetically, Sidney Herbert went on to write that if women selected for nursing in the Crimea did the job creditably, nurses would begin to rid themselves of the reputation for promiscuity and drunkenness that had attached to them in civilian hospitals.

Fortunately for the nurses setting out for the Crimea they were not going to be hindered in their work by lack of money. The public response to *The Times* appeal for a nursing fund had been magnificent and it was put entirely at Nightingale's disposal. Furthermore she did not draw her own allowance of £500 a year from her rich father. It was put into the general fund for medical comforts of her patients. From her own funds she installed laundry boilers in the hospital at Scutari, employed soldiers' wives to do the washing, bought kitchen utensils, brooms, soaps and towels and in doing so made enemies amongst the army medical officers. The truth was that many of them were jealous of the mandate given to her by the government.

In the terms of reference confirming her appointment, the secretary of state for war made it quite clear that she was to have supreme and undivided control of her own nurses. To make everything about her position clear an official appointment was made on 18 October 1854. Florence Nightingale was to have the rank of 'Superintendent of the Female Nursing Establishment of the English General Hospitals in Turkey'.

Such a distinction in army records had never before been placed upon a woman. Her appointment caused a great deal of huffing and sniffing amongst a chauvinistic general staff.

Unfortunately the official designation of her responsibilities carried one flaw. It was, for weeks, going to make her role in the

Crimea almost impossible. The word 'Turkey' attached to the end of her title was going to be used by doctors to limit her authority and restrict her activities in the Crimea.

Florence Nightingale was not usually the sort of woman to be put off by entrenched medical arrogance and officialdom. But when she and her thirty-eight nurses arrived at Scutari she was surprised by the hostility she met at the end of her long voyage. She had suspected there would be some traditional and stubborn male prejudice for her nurses to overcome, but she had never envisaged the strength of professional resentment her arrival did produce.

Nor was she prepared for the sight of the horrific conditions then being endured by the casualties at Scutari. But the woman who bandaged dolls in her childhood, who at seventeen had heard the voice of God calling her to His service as a nurse and had taken the tough training in Germany despite the opposition of her parents was not going to be put off by the antagonism of army medical officers. These were mere obstacles to be overcome with help from God and also from her friend the secretary of state for war, in the pursuit of her true life's work.

# 2 Into the Mouth of Hell

'Calamity unparalleled in the history of calamity.'[1]
Florence Nightingale in a letter to the War Office

The nurses' arrival was disheartening. Absolutely. On 4 November 1854 when the cockroach-ridden mail ship, *Vectis*, anchored off Constantinople in driving rain, gale-force winds battered nurses standing at the ship's rail. Shivering, they waited for the small boat to take them ashore to the ramshackle landing-stage for the Selimiye Kislasi Barracks Hospital. Waiting for them within its warren of yellow walls were hundreds of sick and wounded soldiers straight from the battles around Balaclava.

The nurses were all wearing the same ugly, ill-fitting outfits of grey tweed – 'a dirty-looking dressing-gown sort of dress' (as nurse Martha Clough called it in a letter home), grey worsted jacket, plain white cap, short woollen cloak, and a scarf bearing the only bit of colour in the red embroidered words 'Scutari Hospital'. As they stood at the ship's rail watching the wounded soldiers making their way up the steep rutted track to the hospital, they could have been forgiven for wondering if they had made a big mistake.[2]

The walking wounded helped each other, staggering awkwardly through the thick slippery mud. They were in an appalling state, their bandages and uniforms covered in congealed blood and mud. And there was not much help for them when they finally reached the hospital door. All the beds were full. Ahead of them lay miles of damp, stinking corridors with tiles peeling from the walls and a floor slippery with excrement, described later by the hospital commissioners as a 'sea of sewage'. Rain dripped through the roof and latrines overflowed, flooding the wards.

For the nurses there was not much of a welcome either. Doctors made demonstrably clear their objection to having 'young society ladies' foisted upon them. But there were no such 'ladies' among the party. Florence Nightingale had already foreseen this problem in her selection of nurses. Before setting out on the voyage she made it quite clear that everyone was equal. They would eat together, sleep under the same roof and do the same work. There were to be no favours for those who regarded themselves as 'ladies'. Each one of them would be expected to empty bed pans and perform the most menial of tasks, regardless of her social background.[3]

For their accommodation in the hospital the nurses were given four damp rooms, a kitchen and a small closet, all of which had previously been occupied by three doctors. There were no beds other than the Turkish wooden platforms attached to the walls around each room, no bedding and no facilities for cooking.

Florence Nightingale went down to the main kitchen and came back with a little milkless tea for each one of them and a mind full of awful news.

Asking for furniture would be pointless. There was none in the hospital, not even an operating table. Badly wounded soldiers sat on tubs or lay on old doors without anaesthetic whilst surgeons sawed through shattered bones within sight and sound of the next casualty awaiting attention. It was not until much later when Florence Nightingale herself found screens that men were spared the suffering of their comrades and the ordeals they were likely to undergo themselves.[4]

At that time anaesthetics had only just been discovered and were not in general use. It was a terrifying ordeal for patients in all hospitals to undergo an operation and the butchery in the operating theatre of civilian hospitals had so haunted one young medical student, James Simpson, that he vowed to find a way of relieving the pain of such patients. Whilst doctors in the Crimea were strapping soldiers down before hacking off their limbs, Simpson and two of his friends experimented with inhaling various substances. It was Simpson who suggested they should all three try sniffing deeply from a bottle of chloroform. All three fell asleep. On waking, each of these young men felt delighted with the effects and began using it in operating theatres straight away.

Other surgeons followed their example. At the time when soldiers' arms and legs were being so crudely amputated in 1853, Queen Victoria was given chloroform for the birth of Prince Leopold. The queen approved and everyone else, therefore, was sure to do so. Except military surgeons.

The inspector general of hospitals for the British Expeditionary Army in the Crimea, Dr John Hall, was a prize example. He was a strict disciplinarian remembered for the soldier under his command who died after receiving a flogging of 150 lashes. He positively did not believe in chloroform to ease pain and terror in amputations. Pompously he would assert that it was preferable for a man to 'bawl lustily' as the blade was severing his leg than to 'sink silently into the grave'.[5]

Sometimes surgeons worked by moonlight because there were no candles. Without blood transfusions and the after care of nurses, few survived. Casualties poured in from Balaclava. There *The Times* correspondent, William Russell was in no mood to keep the horrors of Balaclava to himself. Once again he shocked readers with his reports:

> Hundreds of men had to go into the trenches at night with no covering but their greatcoats, and no protection for their feet but for their regimental shoes. The trenches were two and three feet deep with mud, snow and half frozen slush. The dead, laid out as they died, were lying side by side with the living, and the latter presented a spectacle beyond all imagination. Men died without the least effort to save them. The sick appeared to be tended by the sick and the dying by the dying.

Then came news of one of the most awful wartime spectacles ever witnessed. But an official account of the action was never given completely at the time. No one wanted to take the blame.

One report said that at precisely ten minutes past eleven on 25 October 1854, Lord Cardigan, resplendent in his blue and maroon uniform with gold trimmings across his chest ordered nearly 700 men and horses of the Light Cavalry brigade to advance against Russian infantry and artillery waiting in well-prepared defensive positions.

Contrary to all the usages of warfare, what was said to be the finest brigade of Light Cavalry ever to leave Britain charged down the valley into the mouths of the Russian artillery, drawn up ready to fire. On each side of that valley, more Russian artillery gunners and riflemen could not believe their eyes when they saw such a target bunched up under their very barrels. It was sheer madness. Incredulous Russian gunners thought the British must surely have made their riders drunk before they would follow such a madcap course. Twenty-five minutes later it was all over. As *The Times* told its readers in an edition of 14 November 1854: 'At 11.35 not a British soldier, except the dead and the dying was left in front of these bloody Muscovite guns.'

There were some survivors, however, and hundreds of wounded. When the final muster of that Light Brigade was made six hours later, of the 673 riders who took part in the charge, 247 were casualties, 113 of them being killed. In twenty-five minutes, 475 horses perished.

The commander responsible, Lord Cardigan, was apparently unaffected by the tremendous courage of his men and rode back to his yacht where he had a bath, drank a bottle of champagne and went to bed.

The wasteful actions of those days filled the hospital ships carrying wounded back to Scutari. The 300-mile voyage usually took eight-and-a-half days. Seventy out of every thousand of those casualties died on the way, through sheer lack of medical attention. No one then thought of having nurses on hospital ships. That was way into the future.

Nurses who saw stretcher-bearers carrying the battle casualties up the hill track, ankle-deep in mud, were horrified to see how insensitively medical orderlies jolted the wounded as they lay on stretchers, their faces ghastly drawn, groaning mouths hanging open.

In the hospital, wounded soldiers lay packed in corridors alongside hundreds of cholera cases. At one time in the barrack hospital 2,434 patients were crowded together. They lay shivering in blankets soaked with blood and their own faeces. All of them were parched with thirst because there were not even enough cups or buckets to bring water round to them.

When nurses got up each morning they could see what an enormous task lay ahead. They were eager to start. But, though the patients were in desperate need of good nursing care, doctors insisted on using their own inefficient male orderlies. Women nurses were being frozen out. They were forbidden to go into wards unless a doctor had given instructions. Doctors drew together defensively. Women must not trespass on their domain.

Incredibly the imbecility of the army medical system prevented nurses from caring for those wounded soldiers. Some doctors even said to Miss Nightingale, 'You will spoil the brutes.'

Officers then did treat soldiers with utter disdain, as blackguards who had enlisted because they could not do anything else, 'the scum of the earth' according to the Duke of Wellington. They expected men to take pain as part of their lot. From generals down to the lowest soldier, military service had a brutalizing effect. The commander-in-chief, Lord Raglan, had had his arm amputated without anaesthetic at Waterloo and then called out to the orderly carrying his arm away, 'Hey, bring that arm back. There's a ring my wife gave me on the finger.'

That same insensitive attitude to suffering was found in the higher echelons of the medical staff, as evidenced by the inspector general of hospitals, Dr John Hall. He was a great bully of a man, with a chip on his shoulder from being overlooked for promotion, and he resented any suggestion of criticism. Consequently when he was asked to report on conditions in the Scutari hospital he wrote: 'Everything is on a creditable footing.' What he did not say was that he was opposed to having women working as nurses in the hospital.

Junior doctors were fearful of incurring his wrath and complied with his wishes, keeping women out of wards. Regimental doctors at that time were in limbo, technically civilians yet under military orders, who wanted to keep their jobs. Apart from complying with Dr Hall's rules, many junior doctors resented having educated women working with them; intelligent observers judging their professional competence.

Why else were doctors so antagonistic towards those well-meaning nurses? Apparently they thought Miss Nightingale's nurses would cause the same sort of trouble as had soldiers' wives while acting as nurses during the Napoleonic wars. They had brought alcohol into the wards, got drunk and gave sexual relief to men recovering from their wounds of sickness.

Though she was not prepared for such opposition from the doctors, Florence Nightingale was not to be put off easily. At first she gave orders to all nurses that they were not to enter a ward unless told to do so by a doctor. She was determined to show doctors that the women nurses were not going to interfere. It was hard for them to leave soldiers untended when they cried for help, but Florence Nightingale was a strict disciplinarian and forbade her nurses from answering those cries. At the same time she played a cunning game of infiltration.

Her first inroad to the wards was via food and cooking. She made pails of arrowroot and wine for patients and prepared special diets prescribed by doctors for soldiers suffering from cholera and dysentery. She impressed doctors by not allowing any food to leave her kitchen unless accompanied by a prescription. It was a logical progression to feed those who could not feed themselves.

So many casualties were pouring in from Sebastopol that she put all her women to work on something they could do far better than any of the men: sewing. They sewed sacking bags to stuff with straw to use as beds in the barrack room. Those straw beds were laid side by side in whatever space was available in the barrack hospital, lining corridors, in store rooms and hallways. More and more sick and wounded were brought in.

Soon wards were overflowing with muddy and bloody wounded men with hardly any space in which to walk without treading on part of someone's body. Unwashed wooden floors crawled with fleas, bugs, lice and parasitic worms. Men often lay without blankets or pillows, their heads resting on their muddy boots. At one time, over a thousand men were suffering from the diarrhoea of dysentery yet there were only twenty chamber pots.

One catastrophe followed another. On 14 November a hurricane hit the Crimea with such force it uprooted trees, wrecked buildings and blew down marquees housing additional field hospitals. It sank the long awaited large cargo ship *Prince*, which had arrived the previous day with warm clothing for troops. Some of it had been offloaded on to lighters and left to be saturated with rain and sea water in the port, because no one would sign for them. Men were left in misery because no one would take responsibility, even though it could have saved the lives of hundreds of soldiers. The ill-fated army was melting away through rain and disease. By 2 January 3,500 soldiers in trenches before Sebastopol were falling sick through inadequate protection against cold and rain. Russian soldiers wore sheepskin coats and fur caps.

It was the coldest winter in human memory. The losses of Britain's small professional army were appalling. Now newspapers such as the *Morning Post* that had so often called for war, denouncing Aberdeen's diplomacy as appeasement, turned to self-righteous anger, printing reports of men fighting without greatcoats in frozen trenches on the heights around Sebastopol and of the wounded packed into wards filthy with dysentery patients and those with reeking gangrenous wounds. Readers were roused into a seething rage.

By December 1854 the administration of the hospital had almost broken down. Little direction of medical care was evident. The man who should have been in control, Dr Menzies, was recalled to Britain as incompetent. Then gradually it dawned upon the harassed doctors that a remedy was at hand. Competent nurses could bring order out of chaos.

At last doctors at Scutari saw reason and recognized the value of nurses ready to work all hours, and soon they were organizing reasonable nursing care. Florence Nightingale herself, on top of all her administrative work, still spent eight hours a day dressing wounds and caring for patients desperately ill with cholera. She showed complete disregard for contagion and her own safety.

So it was that when another hospital commission investigated the situation at Scutari, most of Miss Nightingale's nurses were fully occupied. At that time, too, more nurses were being mobilized in London under the control of nurse Mary Stanley. But that did not please Miss Nightingale.

A letter on 14 December told her the news. She was furious because she had not been involved in their selection and allocation to hospitals. Furthermore, many of them were Roman Catholic nuns who would owe obedience only to their mother superior, and not to herself as the appointed superintendent. To make matters worse, Miss Stanley had instructions to report directly to the medical director, Dr Cumming, who was to allocate nurses to hospitals as he thought fit. That really was undermining Miss Nightingale's authority. Immediately she wrote a letter to the War Office protesting against having the total control of nurses taken away from her.

It was a bitter controversy, combining the religious fervour of Mary Stanley, jealousy, and the thoughtlessness of a war minister harried by political events. These ingredients led to a period of bickering and open questioning of Florence Nightingale's authority. Charge and counter-charge flew backwards and forwards between Whitehall and Scutari.

When the second party of nurses arrived, all Miss Nightingale's fears about their selection were confirmed. Ten of those 'nurses' were 'ladies' who had never held paid employment in their lives and fifteen were Catholic Sisters of Mercy from Ireland. All of them, she thought, were simply philanthropic women who would be completely out of place in hospitals taking casualties from the Crimea battle-fields.

In fact many of these new arrivals were prepared for hard work and put their lives at risks too, working long hours with the sick and wounded. They were set to work by Inspector General Hall who interpreted literally Miss Nightingale's authority as 'Superintendent of all Female Nurses in Turkey' and therefore not applicable to Balaclava, which was in the Crimea and separated from Turkey by 300 miles of the Black Sea.

Lord Raglan has asked for eleven nurses to be sent to Balaclava hospital, which then was an awful place.

The whole area reeked of death and decomposition. Piles of arms and legs amputated after the battles had been thrown into the almost tideless, lagoon-like harbour, and could be seen in the clear water from the jetty; bodies rose out of the mud and floated to the surface. In parts, the water was covered with a repellent brightly coloured scum. A sulphurous smell of rotten eggs pervaded the whole area.

Despite reports of those conditions some of the newly arrived nurses volunteered to go there in order to escape the discipline of Miss Nightingale. Others went to overflow hospitals established at Koulali, Smyrna and Renkoi. The further from Scutari and the presence of Florence Nightingale that these nurses worked, the more they were appreciated by medical officers. Their competence was quickly recognized at Koulali, for example, whilst at Scutari many surgeons still declined help from women nurses.

Service medical officers were now getting used to the idea of the new wartime nurse.

The Royal Navy employed women nurses at their base hospital at Therapia, established on the Constantinople side of the Bosporos. The Admiralty published a message on 27 November 1854 that read: 'Their Lordships are endeavouring to obtain and send out from England tried and approved female nurses to alleviate as much as possible sufferings and promote the recovery of the wounded.'

Mrs Eliza Mackenzie, 'a lady of experience', and five well-trained nurses arrived to take care of 120 wounded sailors and marines lying in a deplorable state. Unlike Florence Nightingale's reception at Scutari, that of Eliza Mackenzie by naval medical officers was markedly positive. Furthermore the Admiralty made it known that if the experiment at Therapia proved successful, female nursing staff would be established throughout naval hospitals.

Eliza Mackenzie wanted to have some positive experience of nursing before setting off and therefore made several visits to the Middlesex Hospital. The final visit was to witness the amputation of a man's leg above the knee without anaesthetic. It was to be a test of her nerve. She got through the ordeal, for which she had had no preparation, and thereafter felt assured enough to tackle the awesome sights and sounds of a naval hospital in the Crimea.

She set off on Christmas Day 1854, travelling overland with her group of nurses via Marseilles, where they took a French steamer to the Crimea. She arrived at the makeshift hospital, situated in a 'rickety three storey Turkish private house', supervised by Dr David Davidson and staffed by a rag-taggle collection of male orderlies prone to bouts of heavy drinking.

Dr Davidson was delighted to be able to put his new women nurses to work straightaway under Mrs Mackenzie's supervision. All appeared to work smoothly except for some initial bad-tempered disagreements arising from Victorian class distinctions and the fact that the nurses were cramped in their living quarters. Sensibly, Eliza Mackenzie, not wanting to put in jeopardy the long-term prospects for women nurses in the Royal Navy, made sure that staff problems

were kept away from Dr Davidson. She also took care that her
women nurses did not supersede the male nurses.

She also had to deal diplomatically with a backlog of dirty sheets,
which had not been dealt with by Miss Stanley and her nurses – those
turned away from Scutari by Florence Nightingale. She solved the
problem by employing Maltese women to do the washing and
Marines to do the ironing.

As with Florence Nightingale she had to deal with large amounts of
'red tape'. But though not as experienced in nursing as Miss
Nightingale, she was an excellent 'housekeeper' and, moreover, able
to find tactful ways round problems without making a big issue out of
them.

She found that sailors were dying unnecessarily – her husband said
they were being murdered – from being left unattended for days in ships
lying in the harbour at Constantinople. During those winter months
many casualties also suffered from frostbite after standing in water-
logged trenches around Sebastapol. 'I never saw such agony as those men
with frost-bitten feat,' wrote Eliza. 'Amputation was the only cure.'

No drugs were available then to alleviate the intense pain from
cannon-fire wounds. In that naval hospital at Therapia nursing orderlies often had to hold patients down on the beds when they cried out
in pain, filling the ward with demented shouts. But Eliza Mackenzie
soon noted that the gentle demeanour of a female nurse could work
wonders with patients tormented by pain and fear.

Clearly the introduction of female nurses to the naval hospital at
Therapia was a success. It showed what could be done when medical
officers received their new help with cordiality and the nurses themselves tactfully respected those already in positions of responsibility
and did not try to take charge.

All things considered, a precedent had been established.

Out of all the different methods of providing nursing care, there
emerged by the end of 1856 a consensus view that what was needed
by a nation at war was a stable, well-trained nursing corps, not hastily
assembled teams of men on short secondments from their regiments.
Lord Raglan had, for example, in May 1855 written to the War
Office, asking for the formation of a trained corps of hospital orderlies to be sent to the Crimea as soon as possible.

A corps of orderlies did arrive. They were poorly trained and
regarded as unreliable men, preferring nights carousing with alcohol
than tending the needs of wounded patients. They paid little attention to one of the hazards faced by all patients – dirt. In fact, few
people recognized its danger. In the wards and operating theatres,

they were careless about antisepsis. Admittedly, the opportunities for washing were limited and it must be said that it was not just the new orderlies who gave little thought to hygiene. Surgeons, doctors and dressers wore their ordinary clothes or even put on old, stained jackets whilst operating to save their everyday ones. Small wonder that the chances of surviving such surgery was slim. Joseph Lister had yet to convince doctors and surgeons that germs entered wounds from hands, instruments, dressings and even the air of the operating theatre. His use of the carbolic acid spray was still ten years away.

Over Christmas 1854 and into January 1855 the British army suffered casualties not only from Russian attacks but also from exposure and pneumonia. Soldiers without proper winter clothing on the heights above Sebastapol huddled together in sodden trenches trying to stop shivering in the icy winds and drenching rain. Thousands of casualties were shipped back 300 miles to the hospital at Scutari.

Nurses now worked without any breaks for meals, looking after thousands of sick and wounded that filled every available space in the hospital and annexes.

It was then that disaster struck the barrack hospital, into which a further 2,500 men were suddenly packed. Patients were dying with alarming frequency – 42 per cent of all being treated. Not surprisingly, when wounded men were packed alongside those suffering from frostbite, emaciation, dysentery, cholera and typhus, the mortality rate for all casualties in that hospital was bound to rise. Incredibly, however, alarm was not so evident amongst all doctors. Many of them were completely against reform and change of any kind. Bluntly they declared that what had been good enough for Wellington in the Peninsular War was good enough for soldiers in the Crimea. Some even went as far as to say that things would have been far better if the War Office had not sent out a bunch of interfering women who undermined the traditional fortitude and stoicism of the British soldier.

The situation got worse.

Mystifyingly men were dying not just of the wounds and sickness they came in with but also from some horrible fever caught in the hospital – a kind of gaol fever. There were so many deaths that the bodies were taken on open carts and transported to large specially dug holes and thrown in.

All this could be seen. But a far worse peril could not, and it did not come to light until someone noticed that certain beds were 'unlucky'. Patients in them died more often than those in other beds. In the terrible winter of 1855/56, a sanitary commission came from

Britain to enquire into these notorious death beds. Inspectors noticed that near these beds the air was more putrescent and noxious than in other parts of the building. When the wind blew from particular directions a foul smell puffed forth from pipes into the wards.

Sanitary inspectors lifted the wooden floorboards and found a network of broken sewers, choked cesspools, quagmires of decaying filth and rotting, slimy rubbish. One report stated that the water supply to part of the hospital was passing through the carcass of a dead horse.

The situation was, as Florence Nightingale wrote to Sidney Herbert, 'Calamity unparalleled in the history of calamity'. Such was her organizational ability, however, that doctors who had been against her arrival came to be dependent on her. She managed the central control of hospital administration.

Now those nurses previously hindered by hidebound regulations were going to show what they could do when the superintendent of female nurses cut through the restricting red tape of military bureaucracy in that piercingly cold Crimean winter.

With some help from the more co-operative doctors and War Office administrators, Florence Nightingale set about making good the glaring deficiencies of hospital supplies. Basic necessities of cutlery, soap, towels had to be provided, and if the army was unable to supply them, Miss Nightingale found them from funds under her own control. She circumvented official bureaucracy and seldom took no for an answer.

Whilst engaged in all the administrative work she took care to see that a high standard of discipline was maintained among her nurses. No nurse was allowed to walk out of the hospital without being accompanied by the housekeeper or by a party of at least three other nurses.

In order to establish standards of nursing among all hospitals now functioning in the campaign area, Miss Nightingale embarked upon tours of inspection to make sure all achieved a satisfactory level of cleanliness and efficiency. Antiseptics were not yet available, but the guiding principle laid down by Florence Nightingale was to keep everything clean with soap and water.[6]

She never overlooked the needs of the patient himself and especially his requirement for nourishing food. She was fortunate in enlisting the help of a Frenchman famous for his culinary skill, Monsieur Soyer, who at one time had been chef to the Reform Club in London. He it was who invented the field cooking stove with which cooks went to France in 1939. Not only did he help with cooking for patients in Scutari but accompanied Florence Nightingale to the hospitals further east in the Crimea itself.

Soon the effects of her devotion to duty were evident in all hospitals, but there was still much to be done in that bitter winter of 1854/55.

# 3 Order out of Chaos

'The authorities generally treat the Medical Officers with cool disrespect and indifference.'

*The Times*, 1854

In Britain, too, during that January of 1855 the country was having one of the coldest spells of weather in human memory. A freezing fog hung over London when Parliament reassembled and an irate John Roebuck, the radical MP for Bath, demanded a parliamentary committee be set up to enquire into the deplorable mismanagement of the medical provision for the Crimean War.

He had seen for himself how the British army at Sebastapol was losing men at the rate of a regiment a day and how absurdly the nurses were hindered in treating those casualties. There were more men in hospitals than were encamped before the front at Sebastapol. The figures he gave stunned members into silence. Some 12,000 in hospitals, 11,000 at the front! At the same time, newspaper reports of nurses coping with casualties filthy with dysentery and gangrenous wounds, packed into overcrowded, badly equipped hospitals built over Scutari cesspits, aroused a wave of public indignation that brought down the government.

So it was that on 4 February 1855, the ambitious and high-spirited Henry Palmerston was summoned to Buckingham Palace and invited to become prime minister.

He, along with a few diehards, with little regard for the plight of soldiers and nurses in the Crimea, wanted to pursue the war vigorously, to batter the Russian menace into submission once and for all. Times had changed, however. The Russian 'bully', Tsar Nicholas, had died, and the French, who had sent three times as many men as Britain to the Crimea, could see no good reason for fighting Britain's battles and was already suing for an honourable peace.

Despite Palmerston's wish to carry on the war, Parliament had heard enough. Most of them agreed with John Bright's cynical comment that already thousands of Englishmen had died to make 'the unscrupulous' Palmerston prime minister. But as Members debated and scored party political points, nurses in the Crimea worked under ridiculous bureaucratic restrictions that left wounded men suffering unnecessary pain and discomfort, often because medical officers had to abide by the 'proper procedure'. Doctors, well aware of the awful situation, were afraid to report it to higher authority in case they were thought to be 'blowing the whistle' on colleagues and consequently be damned professionally.

Typical of such absurdities was the time when proper clothing for the wounded was 'not available'. Hundreds of wounded soldiers lay without shirts, even when a boat carrying 27,000 of them had arrived, but none could be issued until a proper equipment inventory board had been convened to receive them.

Irritated beyond her patience, Florence Nightingale, like her counterpart Eliza Mackenzie in the naval hospital at Therapia, who was just as exasperated with submitting requisitions in triplicate, found a way round the ludicrous bureaucracy and had several bales of shirts distributed. She saw only too clearly the need for more efficient centralized control of the whole military hospital and nursing system, and she pursued the plan she had already worked out in detail. She sent it to the War Office, with which she still had a privileged relationship allowing direct contact. With War Office support she brought order out of chaos for those wartime nurses.

In that long, marrow-chilling winter of 1855 for which British and French troops were ill prepared, sickness, military skirmishes, and exposure killed thousands of front-line soldiers and rendered thousands more unfit for service. Russian losses were said to be higher still. Morale on both sides sank. Everyone from soldiers to nurses had had enough of war.

It was a particularly distressing time for nurses. Not only were they having to endure personal hardships, they were also being denied the satisfaction of doing their job with adequate facilities to call upon. Florence Nightingale waged one dispute after another with the hierarchy at Scutari.

Another irritating development caused her a good deal of stress. It was the long-running disagreement over who was to be in control of all nurses in the Crimean campaign, as well as the conditions under which they nursed.

It was then that a commission led by Lord Shaftesbury and staffed by eminent doctors and civil engineers was sent to the Crimea with responsibility for making a thorough inspection of all hospital facilities. They were authorized to make any changes deemed necessary without reference to higher authority.

Gradually, with their help, the conditions in Crimean campaign hospitals were greatly transformed. No longer were hospitals muddling through, making do with shortages. Wards were clean and run in an orderly manner; nurses were well disciplined with a strict code of rules to observe.

Supplies for the hospital came through regularly, and the mortality rate in wards dropped from the awful 42 per 100 to 22 per 1,000 – thanks to the insistence on absolute cleanliness.

Patients also were benefiting from more nourishing, appetizing and well-cooked food. Here again it was due to the influence of Florence Nightingale, helped by her French chef, Monsieur Soyer.

Even so Florence Nightingale still lived in the same damp room, into which rain dripped through the roof. She worked long into the night, making her final round of all the mutilated men who lay suffering quietly, row upon row of them, side by side, inches apart. To them all then she was the unforgettable 'Lady of the Lamp'.

Not surprisingly, the long hours of work and the constant bickering with medical and administrative officers took its toll and brought her eventually to a state of physical and mental exhaustion.

Coincidentally the same strain from a demanding workload in a harsh climate at the Royal Navy hospital had undermined the health of Eliza Mackenzie, too, and she was advised by doctors to return home to recover.

The cost of eighteen months of war in the Crimea began to be reckoned. Exactly 19,584 British soldiers had died, and of those deaths fewer than one in ten was due to enemy action. French losses were much higher, 70,000 dying from wounds or disease.

By the end of 1855, apart from a few diehards who detested Russians, people in Britain were now eager for the war to end.

Florence Nightingale, too, was ready to leave the Crimea. After a long period of wrangling over who was to be in supreme control of the nurses in the Crimean war zone, the matter was clarified in a letter from the War Office. It said: 'Miss Nightingale is recognised by Her Majesty's government as the General Superintendent of the Female Nursing Establishment of the military hospitals of the Army. No nurse is to be transferred from one hospital to another, without consultation with her. The Principal Medical Officer will communicate with Miss Nightingale upon all subjects connected with the Female Nursing Establishment.'

At last Miss Nightingale had got what she wanted. But the letter at army command headquarters was of little concern now, because two days earlier a peace treaty had been agreed.

With the Treaty of Paris in 1856 came no tangible fruits of victory for Britain or France. Yet one must not overlook the fact that Russian expansion was contained and another 100 years would pass before her ships appeared in the Mediterranean. For Britain, one important side-effect of the conflict was that it caused the War Department to take a closer look at the horrendous experiences of nurses on active service in military hospitals. Indeed the Crimea experience triggered a new spirit of self-examination in the way the country should prepare for war.

The army had gone to war as if it had learnt nothing since the battle of Waterloo. It was in no way ready to wage a campaign thousands of miles from home against an enemy superior in both numbers and equipment and within easy reach of its own supply lines. The British army emerged resolved to take stock of the lessons learnt from such inadequate planning.

Among the key reforms that grew from this critical investigation were those recommended by Florence Nightingale on the importance of professional nursing care and the insistence on good military hygiene. Through her personal example and those of her colleagues in the Crimea she raised the whole status of the nursing profession and won for the women of Britain the right to enter into a serious and useful military nursing career. This achievement, in defying the conventions of the age, was nothing short of extraordinary.

Opportunities for women to find satisfying employment were few and far between in those middle years of Queen Victoria's reign. A woman's place was in the home looking after large families. Boys of the 'well-to-do' families were sent away to school and university, and bought commissions in the army, while those from poorer backgrounds went out to learn a skill and earn money to help support their large families. Girls from more affluent families learnt to play the piano, draw, dance, paint and do crochet.

Nursing was the great liberator for young women. The idea of choosing nursing as a career became increasingly attractive. Florence Nightingale might have passed into folklore as 'The Lady with the Lamp', visiting the bedside of wounded soldiers, but on her return to England she was still fired with enthusiasm for the establishment of a more efficient nursing profession. She objected strongly to the attitude of the senior consultant at St Thomas's Hospital, Mr South, who once remarked that nurses 'were in the position of housemaids' and that little could be expected from them. Miss Nightingale soon put a stop to that kind of thinking. In 1860 she established the Nightingale Training School for Nurses at St Thomas's Hospital. There, for the first time, nurses followed a comprehensive curriculum for a year, which apart from instruction in the tending of the sick also included ward management, hygiene and technical lectures from the medical and surgical staff. No longer did nurses just 'pick up' their training on the job. They had to learn and were tested. High standards of integrity were expected of them, too, so that when they qualified and took positions in other hospitals they would spread the word, raising standards wherever they were employed. Their names were on the hospital register, no longer 'housemaids' but certificated nurses with high moral standards and technical expertise.

Of course, there were still the same bones of contention between doctors and nurses and the same prejudices to overcome, but progress was made. Florence Nightingale wrote a handbook giving guidance for *The Introduction of Female Nursing into Military Hospitals*.

Florence Nightingale retained her link with the War Office as a general consultant on army welfare until 1872, when the relationship finally came to an end. However, in this period of transition, another woman was particularly active with Florence Nightingale, Jane Shaw Stewart. She too worked zealously, perhaps too keenly for her own good, to improve the status of military nurses.

At that time, women military nurses were employed only in base hospitals of the army, and on wards with at least twenty beds, such as in hospitals at Chatham and Dublin. Gradually new hospitals were built, most notable being the impressive, palatial Royal Victoria Hospital at Netley at which Queen Victoria laid the foundation stone. That was a memorable occasion, and tragic too.

The queen arrived in the royal yacht with a full escort of gunboats and drew alongside a specially built jetty covered in scarlet carpeting. All went smoothly until the queen was about to perform the ritual of actually laying the commemorative stone. A Royal Salute was to mark the occasion, but sadly one gun fired prematurely. It killed two sailors instantly and injured others. Despite this, the ceremony continued.

When the military hospital at Netley was finished, its façade was grand indeed when viewed from Southampton Water, but inside it was not a hospital liked by army nurses or patients. The wards faced north-east and had no view over the water. Instead windows overlook scruffy-looking outhouses and coal bunkers.

Netley, said to be the largest military hospital in the world, with corridors a quarter of a mile in length, tested the endurance of hundreds of trainee nurses for the next 150 years.

Towards the end of the nineteenth century, another era of hospital building began that influenced the establishment of military nurses. The Herbert Hospital at Woolwich was built to a design approved by Florence Nightingale, and later the Cambridge was erected at Aldershot.

Although initially, in all these new army hospitals there was still a hard core of opposition to the employment of women, a compromise was reached. It was agreed that there would be one Army Corps medical orderly for every ten beds and one woman superintendent over six women nurses, one of whom should be designated as 'linen nurse'.

The woman employed as superintendent at Woolwich was Jane Shaw Stewart. That official appointment looked like the harbinger of better things, opening the way for more and more women nurses to enter military hospitals. But it was not to be so simple a transition, despite the fact that two years later Jane Shaw Stewart's name was published on the British Army List as superintendent general of female nurses at the General Hospital at Netley – the first time a woman's name had ever appeared on the list. For the next five years she watched over both Netley and the Royal Herbert General Hospital at Woolwich, but no more female military nurses were appointed.

Suddenly in May 1868, an official enquiry led to her resignation. Little was said in public but the continuous fight against male prejudice culminated in her downfall. The inquiry's report alleged that Jane Shaw Stewart had outbursts of violent temper that led to low morale among nurses and medical orderlies. The breakdown of co-operation affected even medical officers and patients.[1]

Some doctors still objected to nurses accompanying them on their rounds. They seemed to resent the possibility of this new breed of nurses appraising their work critically. These nurses were more articulate and self-confident, qualities stemming from a higher social and educational background than hitherto.

Jane Shaw Stewart furiously condemned the doctors' lack of co-operation in forthright letters to the director general of the Army Medical Department. A counterblast from a civilian doctor, published in the *Lancet*, called the superintendent 'the *bête noire* of the hospital organisation, whose constant interference was heartily disliked by everyone'.[2]

Even nurses ran to doctors with tales of how their superintendent flew into hysterical rages in front of nurses and patients alike. There could be only one outcome. Doctors froze her out. They refused to discuss matters with her.[3] Inevitably Jane Shaw Stewart resigned.

For the next few years the Army Hospital Corps purposefully reduced the influence of women in military hospitals. For example, when the rules governing the Army Nursing Service were revised in 1885, entry into the nursing profession was restricted to those who were prepared to accept control by the director general of the Army Medical Department. The day of the philanthropic lady tending poor wounded soldiers was apparently over.

However, new wars once again showed how valuable these women nurses were. In the latter months of the century, scarcely a year went by without the British army being involved in campaigns in some part of the world.

In many of those campaigns, military nurses accompanied British troops. A team of nurses from Netley was despatched to the Sudan in 1882 to accompany General Wolsley's expedition to relieve General Gordon at Khartoum. During the next five years thirty-five female nurses were posted as official military nurses to India and to Egypt, particularly to Suez, Ismailia, and Wadi Halfa. They served with ambulance companies and hospital ships, conveying the sick and wounded from the Middle East to military hospitals in Britain.

In all of these military campaigns in the East, nurses found themselves once again treating casualties of disease more often than those with gunshot wounds. Outbreaks of cholera and typhoid brought home to senior army officers the risks troops were running. Clearly evident to them, moreover, was the need for more nurses to accompany the expeditionary forces.

It was not going to be an easy passage for the new wartime nurses though. They became engaged in battles against obdurate male prejudice even in that era. Help came from an unexpected quarter – an appeal for a corps of women military nurses to be trained ready for contingencies of war.

A British army Medical Department surgeon, Major Evatt, who had had active service in India and Afghanistan, prepared and distributed in 1885 a pamphlet proposing the formation of a corps of volunteer female wartime nurses prepared to serve alongside the Regular Army Nursing Service in the combat zone of a foreign war. Candidates for this corps would have to be fully trained as civilian hospital nurses and undergo a period of training with the regular army every year.

Evatt knew that efficient hospitals with women nurses were essential in combat theatres of operations. His ideas were confirmed by women such as Sister Janet King, who had served in the Russo-Turkish campaign of 1878 and the Zulu War of 1879-80, in South Africa.

The need for an expansion of the women's military nursing service was proved beyond any doubt very soon by the demands of the costly South African conflict. Nurses with diverse qualifications – from three years of training to those with a first-aid certificate – flocked to serve with the Army Nursing Reserve.

Most of them had enrolled officially as members of the Army Nursing Reserve knowing full well the risks they would be running. And in fact many of them faced danger and death in the discharge of their duties. They simply repudiated all well-meaning regard for their personal safety by commanding officers and asserted their right to share the responsibilities of their country by helping the sick and the dying wherever they might be and whatever the risk. They were prepared to work under the hardest conditions, living on the simplest fare, as they had been warned prior to enlistment by Surgeon Treves. He had spelt out the risks to be faced by the wartime nurse. 'The work of a hospital nurse is hard and dangerous, dysentery and enteric fever are not dainty diseases.'[4] The truth of this warning was brought out early on in the campaign when Sister Stuart Jones died of enteric fever and Sister Rose died of dysentery. They were the first of many to lose their lives in the service of the sick and wounded in South Africa.

The Boer War was the first major war to be fought with modern weapons, bringing an alarmingly high number of casualties; the need for efficient nursing close to the front line was therefore all the more pressing. These new wartime nurses were to acquit themselves admirably.

# 4 Nurses Respond
# to Disasters

'Those nurses don't seem to mind the bullets a bit but carry
on attending the wounded as if they were on the ward.'[1]
Medical Officer on a South African War hospital train.

The nurses who had been so excited at sailing for active service in the
Boer War in sunny South Africa were soon shocked by the reality of
it all – thousands of wounded soldiers flooding into field hospitals.
Never before had there been a war like this one.

Battle casualties differed greatly from all the more recent frontier
skirmishes fought in India or the Middle East, and this war proved to
be on a far more frightening scale than any waged by Britain between
1815 and 1914. It proved to be the longest, costliest and bloodiest.

A nurse in the first draft to Number One General Hospital,
Wynberg, wrote as follows to the *Nursing Record*:

I never saw anything so awful and sad as some of the casualties
brought in from the battlefield. They were all so patient and good.
Many of them had to have operations at once. Men from the Guards
I had known were so awfully altered I scarcely recognised them.
One realizes now what war means and the utter horror of it. No
words can describe how heart-rending it is to see them coming in on
stretchers. One Gordon Highlander with spinal wounds was paralysed in all but his arms yet was as cheery as if he were well and with
such a store of quaint humour.[2]

Casualties were high, especially in the early months of the war.
Within weeks, many more nurses than the War Office had ever imag-
ined were desperately needed. British women responded magnificently.
At last here was the opportunity for them to play a vital part in the war

44

and for them to show what women could do at the heart of the action on a world stage.

From the beginning of the campaign, nurses showed their determination to get as close to the front as possible. Over and over again they exposed themselves to danger, and medical officers were quick to vouch for the way they were able to care for the wounded far more quickly and save lives. 'They have simply proved their right to attend to the wounded wherever they may be found and we consider the present tendency in some parts to restrict the services of Nursing Sisters to base hospitals to be neither just to our soldiers nor to members of the Army Nursing Service,' wrote one regimental medical officer.[3]

Owing to the fluid nature of the war, nurses worked closer to the action than had hitherto been known.

Nurses were now paid a better salary, and naturally under these new pay conditions, staff selection was crucial. It must be said that recruiting procedures were often faulty in the South African War. Not all those selected for nursing duties were able to carry out the tasks required. Some young ladies undoubtedly volunteered less for patriotic reasons than for personal ones – as one nurse put it: 'to see some fun'.

Groups of them were seen in Harrods buying evening gowns and shoes to 'take to the front'. When they arrived in South Africa, matrons looked askance at them. The superintendent of Princess Christian's Hospital in Pinewood, Natal, was particularly critical of the 'good time girls' seen in the hotel, 'smoking cigarettes with most undesirable companions.'[4] They were probably 'fine young ladies' who inspired the limerick writer of the *Sunday Sun* to pen the lines:

> There was a young belle from North Berwick
> Whose conduct was slightly hysteric
> She followed the guns
> And distributed buns
> To the men who were down with enteric.

The overseas adventures of these pleasure-seeking women enraged senior nursing Sisters enough for them to protest to their seniors back home and to South African newspapers. 'The scandal has reached disgraceful proportions in Cape Town, says the *Empire*. The city is infested with nurses whose zeal outruns their discretion and with women who are nurses only in name. Idle society women have invaded the principal coast towns. Lord Kitchener sent them home after their many mad pranks.'[5]

Wounded servicemen sometimes complained about the 'butter-flies', as they were sometimes called. One patient became so angry with one of these ladies that he wrote to the press: 'These untrained females – fine lady nurses – are no good at all. All they do is sit on an officer's bed and flirt. One ass, posing as a ministering angel with Parisian gown and headgear, muddled about for a week with my arm until at last I gave her a good blowing up and she never came near me again.'[6]

Such comments make it easier to understand the attitude of the small minority of medical officers who were still averse to having women nurses in the traditionally man's world, close to the front. However, once real, fully trained nurses were at work serving regiments close to the fighting, most doctors recognized without reservation how many lives were saved by female professional nurses. One doctor who had seen them at work close to the front line wrote reassuringly to readers back home: 'Nurses are giving excellent service rendering skilled help to the wounded from the front at an early stage, preventing the occurrence of complications which result so quickly when trained nursing is not available.'[7]

When the number of casualties increased alarmingly as the war progressed, the army high command was worried to note that more men were dying from disease than from gunshot wounds. Nurses and doctors were appalled at the general standard of sanitation in hospitals. They realized that stronger measures would have to be taken to prevent disease. Infected dust penetrated everywhere, flies were a menace, there were too many veldt sores (small cuts which became infected) and soldiers too often drank impure water.

Before setting out on a march each man was given a full bottle of clean water, but after marching in hot sunshine, with temperatures rising to 115°F, the bottles were soon emptied. With the usual mode of combat – guerrilla warfare – demarcation lines of battle were not clear, causing difficulties in transporting clean water to troops. Consequently soldiers, ravaged by thirst, filled their bottles from stagnant pools and muddy streams from which animals had been drinking.

By the time the war ended, statistics would show the problem with startling clarity. Of the 22,000 men the British army lost in the South African wars, two-thirds died of disease. Sadly, it was the Crimean experience revisited.

Getting suffering soldiers to hospitals from battlegrounds that changed frequently was a common problem and often brought tragic results. Hospital trains were often attacked on their way down to base hospitals, but reports told of nursing sisters who went on calmly dressing wounds. 'Miss de Montmorency and Sister Rose Innes, taking casualties down from Graspan to Cape Town, are two of the pluckiest women alive,'[8] reported one officer commanding an ambulance train.

Wherever nurses worked, apart from base hospitals, their meals were scanty and barely nutritious. One nurse who went down with enteric fever recorded her diet in a diary. It comprised mainly watery chicken soup, cornflour pudding and small drinks of milk supplied by a local Boer farmer. She recovered but thereafter swore never again to take soup or cornflour pudding.

Such was the demand for nurses that calls were made on the resources of Canada, Australia and New Zealand. Eighty women nurses from various parts of the British Empire responded to the call and served in South African hospitals. Most of them got on very well together, but British nurses had one minor irritation. Canadian nurses had hardly started active service with the British force when they were given the rank and allowances of army lieutenants. Added to their comparatively high pay and officer status was another enviable factor. They were issued with an attractively smart military uniform, comprising short khaki 'bicycling skirt', blouse with epaulettes worn with brown leather belt, boots and an English army nursing service cap.

British army sisters were not granted military rank, though they were generally regarded as having the status of officers. Their uniform was far less practical and attractive than the Canadian. British skirts were long and uncomfortable in very hot weather and completely impractical during the rainy season, when nurses had to live and work in muddy, tented hospitals close to a changing front line.

More often than had been planned, nursing sisters had to work in scantily equipped mobile hospitals that moved with divisions in action. The 'stationary hospitals' – a misnomer in the case of South Africa – were small though adequately equipped with four nursing sisters allotted to each. Casualties would progress from these to the base hospitals, generally sited close to the ports. In each of these hospitals, twenty nursing sisters tended patients before they went back to their units or were evacuated to the United Kingdom.

In the first disastrous months of the war, the Boers invaded Natal and Cape Colony, invested the townships of Kimberley and Mafeking, defeated British forces at Nicholson's Neck and drove the remaining British troops and their nurses back into Ladysmith to which they then laid siege.

Life in Ladysmith for everyone, including nurses, grew more fear-some everyday. In a letter home one nurse wrote:

Shelling once went on for a whole week without stopping. During the bombardment one British officer had to go out with a white flag to ask if the wounded could be removed to a place of safety. We were allowed to remove many of them to a tented hospital set up at Intombi, two and a half miles out of Ladysmith. Marquees were erected on a piece of land which was like a swamp surrounded by hills on which Boer guns were sited. The gunners were so near we could see them smoking pipes and preparing food. All shells fired by them into Ladysmith had to go over our tents. As food became scarcer we managed on a quarter of the rations and our water was rationed each day.

It was hard to keep looking cheerful under such conditions but one had to for any depression on our part was at once communi-cated to the patient and quickly spread around the ward. Fortunately the Red Cross managed to get some provisions through to us. Civilian orderlies had been commandeered from 'superior men' such as the station master and clerks who could be relied upon to do the right thing.[9]

The way nurses went about their duties did much for morale in besieged Ladysmith, as a medical officer later reported. 'Women, when shells were bursting on the ground, crossed the streets as calmly as if no cannon were within a hundred miles,' wrote one astonished officer wishing to convey his admiration to the public back home. And it was the same story in besieged Mafeking until General Baden-Powell brought its relief.[10]

British forces sent to relieve Ladysmith were, in one infamous black week of 10 to 15 December 1899, humiliated by defeats at Stormberg, Magersfontein and Colenso. Casualties poured into under-staffed field hospitals. To the surprise of British commanders, the Boers were using new rifles and artillery imported from European countries many of which were openly in sympathy with the Boers. New breech-loading rifles from France and Germany, with smaller bores, were more accurate, fired more rapidly and could wound at greater distances than older ones used by the British. Furthermore, the Boers were experimenting with a variety of relatively light machine-guns such as the automatic Maxim that could inflict terrible casualties on forces making frontal attacks in extended order.

Another new weapon with which Boers terrified nurses and

patients in British hospitals and wrought havoc on infantry assembling for attacks was 'Long Tom' – a 30-foot-long siege gun that could toss a 40-pound shell four miles with impunity, for it far outraged any retaliating British 15-pounder gun. The 26th Field Hospital, beside the military camp at Dundee, Natal, experienced its devastating potential.

It made no difference to Boer gunners that the 26th Field Hospital flew a 12-foot-high Red Cross flag, so recently accepted at the international Geneva Convention as an indicator of non-combat medical troops. Long Tom's shells crashed down in broad daylight on the hospital tents. It was a distressing sight. Heavily bandaged soldiers crawled out of the debris dragging broken legs, some shuffling on their backs unable to stand, all trying desperately to get away from the area.[11]

On another occasion, the 18th Field Hospital, which housed its wounded in the town hall, received a direct hit from Long Tom (the Boer's long-range gun with the long barrel) that killed ten patients and badly wounded doctors and nurses. According to their commander, Major Donegan, so demoralized was the staff after the shelling that many soldiers, including one doctor, took off into town and drank themselves stupid.

No matter how much care was taken, patients and several sisters died from enteric fever and dysentery. The roll of nurses who lost their lives in the cause of the South African war grew longer each week. One angry nurse wrote home describing the frustrations of a colleague who needed officer rank to get things done:

> Here it is seething with enteric and dysentery and the Sisters and nurses are doing splendid work. Water is so short for washing that many of our patients are covered in pediculi (lice infestation) and nurses do not escape their attentions. It is very disheartening that we cannot do for our patients all we would wish and my experience of male orderlies in military hospitals is best left unsaid. The truth is that nursing does not rank. Many military doctors don't grasp that it exists. There will be a fine battle royal before military medicine realizes the evolution of the art. Meanwhile we muddle on.[12]

Thousands of wounded men needed the best possible professional nursing care to get them fit again to return to their units at the front. It made good sense to have well-qualified women nurses staffing field hospitals as close to the front line as possible. A more efficient medical evacuation service was also needed to get wounded from the battlefield to field hospitals.

The British army was operating over a vast expanse of South Africa, but there were no motor ambulances then. Ox-drawn wagons were used rather than horse-drawn, because with their longer wheelbase they gave casualties a smoother ride as they travelled over the stony veldt.

Back at the railhead, the new hospital trains were ideal. Taking pride of place was one named *The Princess Christian*, in acknowledgment of the help the army nursing service had received from Queen Victoria's third daughter. Each train had accommodation for two nursing sisters and two medical officers.

But there was also a desperate shortage of stretcher-bearers willing to brave enemy fire to rescue the wounded. The deficiency was rectified in a remarkable way.

When General Buller applied to the War Office for more stretcherbearers, he got nothing. In a flash of inspiration he sought help from Natal's Indian community. It was led then by a 28-year-old barrister, a man with a reputation for getting things done. One day he would lead the Indian National Congress in its struggle for national independence. In 1899, though, this pacifist merely wished to show India's loyalty to the Empire. He was Mahatma Gandhi.

As pacifists (in accordance with their Hindu religion), the Indians were unable to fight, but they were willing to act as stretcher-bearers.

So it was that on 15 December 1899 at the camp at Frere, the doctor in charge of the 4th Field Hospital, Dr Treves, witnessed a strange procession. Some 2,000 volunteer stretcher-bearers marched ahead of their field hospitals towards the battle line. With the 800 Indian volunteers were a further 1,200 'body snatchers', as cynical troops called them, that General Buller had recruited from refugees who had fled Johannesburg.

Dr Treves lingered at the front of his tent as another small squad of men approached, singing a coarse song about the dead and the dying. They were a burial party of private soldiers who had learnt by the brutalizing effect of war to hide their true feelings behind a screen of tobacco smoke and gallows humour.

The doctor in charge of that field hospital was probably the last medical specialist one would expect to see in the desolate war-torn veldt of South Africa, for Dr Treves was the queen's surgeon. He was learning something new every day.

What he saw in the next few days, though, appalled him.

He had set up his field hospital a little way behind the front line. Once again it was evident that British commanders had still not learnt lessons from earlier frontal attacks on Boer positions manned by sharpshooters and rapid-firing machine-gunners. The consequences were catastrophic.

Dr Treves watched processions of stretcher-bearers staggering over stony ground and buffeting their loads of groaning men – men he had watched striding forth in the early morning singing. Now they were burnt fiery red by the sun, and covered in dust and sweat. Their army shirts were stiff with dried blood. Treves, a man used to the sight of blood and terrible accidents, felt his stomach heaving. The men were lying delirious; sometimes they rolled off the stretchers. The earth seemed to be covered by men tormented by the pain of fly-blown wounds (those upon which bluebottles or blowflies had laid their eggs which then developed into maggots).

That evening when the sun went down, rain fell continuously. Orderlies attempted to cover men lying outside tents on stretchers, with tarpaulin sheets. Those close to the surgeon's operating tent shuddered as they heard what was happening inside, despite the orderlies' calming words: 'Don't worry, mate. You won't feel a thing.'[13]

At least those soldiers on the makeshift operating tables tended by army surgeons and volunteer nurses had the merciful benefit of chloroform denied to men of the Crimea War, whose sawn-off limbs were thrown into buckets outside the tent.

At Intobi there were only fifteen nurses to look after 1,400 wounded soldiers. Inside the besieged town of Ladysmith three hospitals – the 11th, 18th and 24th – handled over 10,000 casualties between November 1899 and the end of February 1900. 'To use an overworked comparison,' wrote one nurse in her diary, 'it was like Hell on Earth.' A typhoid epidemic raged. Food and medical comforts were in short supply. Some 500 men died.

Of the nursing sisters tending the wounded in the besieged Ladysmith, a serving chaplain wrote in his book, *Chaplain at the Front*:

It was a marvel of heroic endurance for gentle women to live in a camp exposed to wind and rain and cold, almost perpetually on duty, each with some sixty patients under her care and most of them in a dying condition; whilst their food was unpalatable and barely sufficient to satisfy their hunger. In their devotion they sacrificed years out of their lives to give comfort to "Tommy". Truly, without exception they were all worthy of the Royal Red Cross medal.

The death rate at Bloemfontein was even worse. Ten men were dying every day, and wagons drawn by mules took their grim loads of bodies, sewn into blankets, down the main street, accompanied by token escorts of soldiers with rifles carried in the funeral drill position of 'arms reversed'.

The neglect of sanitary precautions that Florence Nightingale had insisted upon forty years earlier was scandalous. The gruesome picture was described by William Burdette Coutts in a report to *The Times*: 'So pitiful was the condition of the wounded. They lay on the stony ground on nothing more than thin waterproof sheets with hardly any food, the dying alongside those wounded but still alive.'

The Boers were elusive. They moved rapidly from one front to another. Every farmhouse in the country was supplying food and shelter to small fighting groups of mounted riflemen who harassed an army at first too small for effective operations over so vast a field. The Boers' tactics were to inflict maximum losses on British units and retire quickly under cover of night and so live to fight another day at a place of their choice. In this kind of warfare nurses were always at risk.

These 'hit and run' tactics caused commander-in-chief General Roberts to take stern measures. He was told to treat the guerrillas simply as bandits. With such arguments prompting him, and senior officers urging him on, Roberts took violent reprisals. He had little sympathy with the Boers anyway, for they had killed his son, Lieutenant Roberts, at Colenso, and he had few scruples about instigating another harsh policy: setting fire to Boer farms.

His troops seemed to enjoy this task. One report from Private Bowers tells how his platoon was in a Boer farm spending a pleasant evening singing around the piano, when they just decided to pile up all the furniture and set fire to the whole farm. Bowers claimed that all units were doing the same thing. 'The idea was to starve the Boers out,'[14] he said.

Even *The Times* leader writer approved such barbaric acts. 'The guerrillas must be taught a lesson by retaliatory measures.'[15]

The burning of farms and slaughtering of livestock became a deliberate anti-guerrilla strategy of destroying homesteads that provided intelligence and supplies to Boer commandos. Thus a new and more terrifying kind of war developed, a war in which military nurses often found themselves under fire. The Boers struck viciously at British units where hospitals were exposed and nurses often felt the brunt of hit-and-run attacks. The war now knew no rules.

British trains were derailed. By moving swiftly across the countryside Boer guerrillas caused widespread devastation along British lines of communication, leaving a frightening number of casualties, amongst them many nurses, especially those on hospital trains. Twenty-four of them died on active service. Roberts's successor, Lord Kitchener, pushed the farm-burning strategy to the limit, ordering the burning of 30,000 republican farms. Troops swept the country burning any place that would sustain Boer guerrillas. They took women and children from their homes and flung them into the nearest of twenty-four concentration camps set up for the purpose.

For each camp in which women and children were concentrated, one doctor and a handful of nurses were allocated. Rations were set deliberately near starvation level so as to 'encourage' guerrilla men to give up the struggle through feeling pity for their families. It was a diet on which typhoid could thrive. Kitchener did not seem to care at all about this risk, even though children were the first to go down with the disease. He never visited one of the camps, saying there were more important matters for him to deal with. He lied in his reports to the War Office, saying of the gruesome camps that 'Everything is under control and the inmates are very happy.'

Official estimates vary on the numbers who died. Of the 200,000 interned, between 18,000 and 26,000 died of typhoid, dysentery, measles, malnutrition and other camp diseases.

Many were the lessons, medical and strategical, to be learnt from those ghastly and brutal South African wars. After its early defeats and an outbreak of cholera, the army accepted 3,000 male orderlies. Unfortunately male nursing orderlies were frequently found to be inept and callous, and were often suspected of stealing from their comrades.

Patients were often afraid of them, yet dared not complain. They even feared telling visiting inspectors about their abuse by male orderlies, because of being bullied later. One trumpet major patient, for example, said in a subsequent court of inquiry into complaints against Army Hospital Corps orderlies: 'I did not complain of these things to the visiting officers because when Gunner Lester reported George the orderly, he threatened to jump on his stomach and stamp his lights out.'[16]

Regularly *The Times* printed lurid accounts of the filth and neglect in hospitals, shortage of medical stores and food. War correspondents pressed for more fully qualified female military nurses. Support for this policy came from Alfred Keogh, director general of Army Medical Services, who said of nurses in South Africa: 'Their importance to efficiency is greater than they know.'[17]

Further unstinted praise came from medical officers who had worked with well-qualified military nurses in South Africa for the first time. One aspect gained particular approval. A nurse herself expressed it in a letter to the *Nursing Record*: 'One thing we have all decided; and this is, that in future wars both hospitals and women nurses must be carried nearer the front. Women would not be murdered or ill-treated – in a white man's land any more than the sick and wounded are.'

Towards the end of the South African wars senior commanders came to realize that good nursing was crucial to military efficiency, as was an expanded female nursing service. At this time, too, help came from the royal family. The Princess of Wales, later to become Queen Alexandra, herself enlisted a large contingent of nurses from the staff of the London Hospital, for service in South Africa.

For the Boer War, Britain committed a quarter of a million men and more military nurses than ever before. When the war began on 11 October 1899, there were only eighty nursing sisters trying to cope with a catastrophic number of casualties. By the end of the war, 1,400 women nurses were serving in twenty-two general hospitals, each with over 500 beds. Nurses had indeed proved themselves as an essential part of wartime medical care.

But to meet the demands of even bigger conflicts that some already saw looming on the horizon, provision would have to be made quickly to expand the nursing service before hostilities began.

Looking back over that turbulent half century beginning with the Crimean War, we can see that the War Office forced a female nursing service on the army, simply because women nurses proved themselves better than their male counterparts.

After the South African wars recruiting for good nurses began in earnest at a time when few career opportunities were open for women. The army could thus choose to be discriminating in those they selected. Women had to complete three years' training in a civilian hospital, followed by a further six months' rigorous probationary service at the military hospital at Netley.

Even with improved pay and conditions, nursing was still essentially a 'labour of love'. There were few promotion prospects as an incentive for nurses to volunteer for military service. Civilian hospitals provided far more opportunities for gaining experience in a wider variety of cases and the chance to use more up-to-date equipment. Furthermore an experienced civilian nurse could command a much higher salary as a civilian matron than as a superintendent in the army nursing service.

Gradually too at this time, the feeling grew among women nurses that those who risked their lives and health in war zones should at least have their combatant status clearly defined, like the rest of the army. Moreover, military nurses wanted commissioned rank in order to control their orderlies.

Support for their cause came from Queen Victoria herself. She informed the War Office, too, that she wanted an award for distinguished service by women nursing sisters – twenty-four army nurses had lost their lives in South Africa. So it was that a royal warrant created the Royal Red Cross for special devotion to duty and professional competence.

One of the first recipients of the award was Eleanor Laurence. She served as a nurse with the army in the Boer War and achieved the distinction of a civilian nurse, being awarded both the Royal Red Cross and the South African War Medal in 1901 for gallantry under enemy fire.

Mention should be made too of another nurse who distinguished herself at that time. Mrs Grimwood's heroism was recorded in India, when under heavy fire she was trying to alleviate the suffering of the wounded during the siege of the Residency at Manipur. An account of her bravery in the *Nursing Record* of 11 June 1891, said she had done more than enough to be awarded the Victoria Cross.[18]

However, despite the steady recognition of their worth, military nurses still remained in a subordinate position and with an uncertain status within the army medical service. It was time that the whole of the Army Nursing Service came under a radical review, and the man to do just that had recently been appointed director general of Army Medical Services – Alfred Keogh. He drew up a comprehensive program based on lessons learnt in the recent conflicts.

The great step forward for military medical officers and nurses came on 23 June 1898, when by a royal warrant the Royal Army Medical Corps was formed. In recognition of its independence it was given its own badge and a motto, *In Arduis Fidelis* (faithful in adversity). To distinguish members of the corps from other regiments, its uniform bore a dark red facing.

Looking forward to wars of the future, Keogh predicted that casualties would be so heavy that optimum use must be made of both men and women. In any case, he reasoned, all able-bodied males would have to be available for front-line duties. Therefore, women nurses would have to be given a permanent place in the planning for war. To this end in 1901 army nursing sisters were placed on the war establishment of the medical services. Then, on 27 March 1902, the new Queen Alexandra's Imperial Military Nursing Service (QAIMNS) replaced by royal warrant the Army Nursing Service.

It too had its own badge, whose concept was chosen by Queen Alexandra – the cross of Dannebrog from her native Denmark, worn on the right side of the scarlet cape, worn over a grey dress.

Furthermore, prospects for a career in military nursing were greatly enhanced by a reorganized structure. The QAIMNS was given a new and extended hierarchy comprising a matron-in-chief, principal matron, sister and staff nurse. The service doubled in strength and salaries were raised to a level above those for civilian sisters and staff nurses. Special leave on full pay was to be granted for in-service training in civilian hospitals.

In 1908 the QAIMNS Reserve was formed and in the same year a Territorial Army Nursing Service came into being. In the few years before 1914 the First Aid Nursing Yeomanry (FANY) was also expanding as a military ambulance movement. Added to these movements on the eve of the war was the Voluntary Aid Detachment for which 50,000 women enrolled. Armed with qualifications in first aid and home nursing they were trained to nurse under field conditions and earned praise from veteran matrons of the QAIMNS.

Thus by 1914 a more efficient army nursing service was ready for what was soon to be called the 'Great War'. It was a conflict that would take nurses not only to France but all over the world, from the Arctic winters of Archangel through Italy, Serbia, Macedonia, Greece, Turkey, Mesapotamia, and Africa. They would care for an appalling number of casualties – four times as many men would be killed in action as in the Second World War – and nurses would show themselves to be as heroic as men in the casualty clearing stations, ambulance service and hospitals. In such faraway places, 200 nurses would lose their lives in military service. As the historian H.A.L. Fisher was later to write: 'Every record for valour previously established was here surpassed.'[19]

# 5 The Challenge

'It was after football, when he'd drunk a peg,
He thought he'd better join. – He wonders why,
Someone had said he'd look a god in kilts,
That's why; and maybe too, to please his Meg:
Ay that was it, to please the giddy jilts
He asked to join. He didn't have to beg:
Smiling he wrote his lie, aged nineteen years.'[1]
From 'Disabled', Wilfred Owen

It was a bright June afternoon in 1914 when Sister Mayne went into the tea room of the hostel for young women at Newington Causeway. Immediately she was struck by the excited hubbub of talk, all the more noticeable because of the variety of languages: English, French, German, Norwegian, Swedish, Dutch and Danish.

Someone had shot the heir to the Austrian throne and his wife.

But as summer days went by, heatwaves, thunderstorms, new autumn fashions, the latest ragtime hits, the county cricket league table and the threat of civil war in Ireland were the topics that dominated conversations and newspaper headlines. Few journalists then seemed to think that the shooting of the little-known Franz Ferdinand would destroy the stability of Europe.

But the shots at Sarajevo, Bosnia, did spark off the Great War of 1914-18, though its origins lay more in the rivalry between European nations, looking to expand or protect their empires. At that time in 1914, Bosnia-Herzogovina had been taken within Austria-Hungary's boundaries. The people in those newly acquired territories were hostile to the rule of the old Austrian emperor, Francis Josef, and it was in the hope of regaining some popularity that the Austrian government thought it wise to stage a royal procession through the streets of Sarajevo. The archduke hoped that a show of military power would subdue rebellious factions wanting to be reunited with neighbouring Serbia. The royal celebrities chosen for the procession were the heir to the throne himself, Franz Ferdinand, Archduke of Austria, and his wife Sophie.

At ten o'clock on that sunny Sunday morning, which incidentally was the feast of St Vitus, thousands of Bosnians were milling through the streets in a festive holiday mood. Among them were six teenage Bosnian nationalists, sworn to kill Franz Ferdinand.

As the procession of royal cars drove slowly through the crowded streets, one assassin threw a bomb. It missed the archduke but wounded his colonel, who was rushed to a military hospital. Then Franz Josef's car drove quickly to receive a loyal welcome from the mayor of Sarajevo, before speeding back to the hospital to visit the colonel. The driver took a wrong turning.

'Stop!' shouted the military governor in the car. The driver braked abruptly and wrestled with the heavy steering. At that moment two Bosnian fanatics saw a chance to have another go at Franz Ferdinand. One of them, Gavrilo Princip, barged through the crowd and fired his pistol twice. The first shot killed the archduke and the second his wife.

Events then moved swiftly. On 21 July Austria presented an ultimatum to Serbia. Serbia made a placatory reply, which Austria did not accept, and on 28 July she declared war on Serbia.

It was at this time that the young European women staying with Sister Mayne at the Newington Causeway hospital began making a frantic rush for the ferryboats to take them home.

At the same time diplomats all over Europe swung into action. They talked, negotiated, and even pleaded, but seemingly unstoppable forces were driving everyone to war. War fever swept Europe. Strangely enough, the prospect of war seemed to fire the men and women of Britain with a sense of adventure. Young men were proud to be British.

'There was a great sense of patriotism throughout the country. I remember it well,' recalled Wilfred Taylor, who served in the Royal Army Medical Corps. 'Whenever the national anthem was played at the end of a variety show we'd stand to attention and sing all the words too whilst the musicians in front of the stage tried to keep up with the audience.'

Sister Jean Robson, who had been nursing in Huddersfield Fever Hospital, recalled the same feeling of excitement in the air.

Even during a theatre performance a tremendous surge of emotion went through us all whenever the female star of the show came on, regaled as a guardsman in a tight figure-hugging uniform, and marched round the stage singing the old South African war songs of "We're the soldiers of the Queen, me lads who've been my lads, who've seen my lads ..." Later on, some theatres even held special recruiting nights, with wounded soldiers brought onto the stage as the band played the popular hit song: "We don't want to lose you but we think you ought to go ... We shall cheer you, thank you, kiss you, When you come back again." Young lads and married men left their seats and formed up on the stage. That's the way it was then. A few came back.

Suddenly the stark reality of it all hit the nation. On 1 August 1914 Germany declared war on Russia, and on 2 August German troops marched into Luxembourg and into Belgium on 4 August. At 11 p.m. on that same day, Britain declared war on Germany. All the vague talk about squaring accounts with the Kaiser became a reality that would touch everyone at home.

After days of doubt the certainty of war brought a kind of excited resignation that could be seen on people's faces. It was in this atmosphere that the QAIMNS, in common with the fighting services, made ready for action.

A poster was distributed, showing the baleful war minister General Kitchener pointing his finger at the reader above the words: YOUR KING AND COUNTRY NEEDS YOU. The effect was immediate – 100,000 men volunteered overnight. Enlistment was for three years. Few had planned for as long as that. They had thought it would all be over by Christmas.

Boys eager to join men in uniform falsified their ages to enlist. Typical of these boys keen to fight for their country was sixteen-year-old William Hunter, a cabin boy who jumped ship in Montreal, made his way back to Liverpool, and joined the Loyal North Lancashire Regiment. Likewise, Joseph Byers was just sixteen when he joined up on 20 November 1914; two weeks later he was on the boat to France. Herbert Burden, too, was only sixteen when he joined the 1st Battalion of the Northumberland Fusiliers.

Little could they imagine that their names would be the centre of discussion in Prime Minister Blair's cabinet room in 1999, as we shall see. Boys and young men all over Britain in 1914 rushed to join up to get into action before the war ended.[2]

In draughty old buildings throughout the country, medical examination rooms were set up. Men stripped off in acute embarrassment and coughed while doctors felt around their groin for signs of hernia.

Volunteers bristling with eagerness took the ritual in good part. A joke of the time ran, 'The doc looks into your ear and if he doesn't see daylight from the other side, you're in.'

Finally those who passed the medical exam gathered in another room and took the oath of loyalty. Once they accepted the king's shilling there was no going back.

Nurses were not immune to the excitement. Young women with some nursing experience volunteered in greater numbers than ever before. Territorial and reserve nursing sisters were called to their respective military hospitals, where they were inoculated against enteric fever and prepared for service in whatever part of the world they were needed. With sore and swollen arms, many with aching heads too, they brought their uniform and kit up to field service readiness.

At the War Office, Dame Ethel Becher was in charge of administration of the nursing service, and preparing nurses for embarkation. Each nurse received an identity disc bearing name and religion. Few recipients realized then their grim significance. They thought they had something to do with attendance at church parades.

In August 1914 there were scarcely 300 nurses in the QAIMNS, but within four months they numbered 2,223 and by the end of the war 10,404 had enrolled. In addition to those nurses available in 1914 there were also almost 9,000 members of the Voluntary Aid Detachments ready to work on the wards as assistants to the trained nurses. By the end of the war there would be 23,000 of them.

Sister Mayne and her colleagues in the QAIMNS got their posting orders straight away. One of the first things she did was to take off her wedding ring. She dashed into a post office, took two pieces of blotting paper from the writing desk to disguise the shape of the ring, and slipped it into a registered envelope and addressed it to her husband Gerald. She had already written to say she was going to France.[3]

Dressed in her travelling cloak, ankle-length dress and grey bonnet, tied with a bow under the chin, she arrived in France with the first contingent of nurses on 12 August 1914. In direct control of all nurses with the British Expeditionary Force was Dame Maud McCarthy of the 1st General Hospital.

Everything for nurses was smoothly organized. Sister Dorothy Hay, who soon would serve in Serbia, wrote in her diary: 'Everything was done in such a rush and yet was so well organised as if our call up for war had been long expected and plans worked out to the last detail.'

Sister M.B. Peterkin, with a few colleagues of the QAIMNS

reserve bound for the 9th General Hospital, left Edinburgh's Waverley Station at 10.50 p.m. on 11 August, travelled through the night and arrived in London at 7.30 a.m. They were taken immediately for breakfast at the Ladies' Club and instructed afterwards to go to the tailor's for their military uniforms and buy anything else they might need in France. 'Rushing about from one shop to another in that boiling hot August was not my idea of enjoyment,' she wrote in her diary. But there was to be no rest for those nurses.

We had to report to Fort Pitt hospital for a medical examination, inoculation – the typhoid was optional but most of us took it. We were roused at 4.50 a.m. for the train at a Rochester siding. We felt very seedy with the effects of our inoculation and lack of sleep but by mid-day we were staggering up the gangway of an Anglo-Canadian trooper. It was a South American cargo ship converted for troop-carrying duties.

That night they sailed to Le Havre, disembarked in the cold wet dawn and were taken on familiar London buses to a train bound for Rouen. The British army was so short of transport that they had bought old B-type buses, covered the red and cream paint with dull grey and boarded up the windows. Each bus could then carry twenty-five fully equipped soldiers. Drivers were organized into auxiliary omnibus companies and played a vital role in moving British divisions on the Western Front.

On the train, nurses were packed eight to a compartment but it was at least some consolation for them to know they were more comfortable than soldiers who sprawled on their kit-bags in goods train box-cars marked 'Hommes 40 Chevaux 8' (Men 40, Horses 8). As the train drew out of the station soldiers stood by the open doors neighing like horses. War was still an amusing adventure.

All night it rained.

It was a long tiring journey, with the train stopping and dawdling along the line, all through the night. Never had those nurses been so pleased to see a superior as they were when dawn broke and a smartly dressed, senior matron opened their compartment door. She told them to get off the train and into transport waiting for them. Again the 'transport' was surprising.

There was a row of shop delivery vans [recalled Sister Peterkin] with addresses of London and Glasgow on their sides. We were bundled into them and taken to the Convent of St Madelaine. The

rooms were very small and there was no space to walk between our
beds. We ate in a rough hotel nearby. The food was awful but at least
hot and that was really appreciated for although it was August the
cold rain came down incessantly. Everywhere seemed damp and
cold.

Within a few days of the mobilization of nurses, military hospitals
were established close to the British Expeditionary Force (BEF). On
22 August 1914 the British army completed its concentration near
Mauberge on the Belgian frontier near Mons. The next day, 23 August
1914, six German divisions attacked the two British divisions, which
fought desperately to hold the line. After losing 1,600 men to superior German firepower British divisions retreated in some disarray.
Many of the 'walking wounded' found themselves retiring on their
own or in small groups.

Astonishing reports tell how one of those groups, cut off by the
speed of the German advance in the fighting at Mons, turned in
horror to see Germans with fixed bayonets and some cavalry charging upon them. Then a miracle happened. Or so it was universally
believed at the time. A platoon of angels was said to have intervened.[4]

Two British nurses, Sisters A. and R. McGuire, then with the BEF,
described the incident in a letter to their cousin in the United States.
'Just as our men turned to meet certain death on the charging
German bayonets, a troop of angels appeared on the battlefield and
stood between them and the Germans. Our soldiers saw them quite
plainly and how the German horses took fright, like Balaam's ass of
old, and our men had time to get away.'[5]

Authenticity was given to this account by a letter in *The Dispatch*
from Canon Marrable, who knew two officers in the group. Another
man of the church, Canon Willinkes of Birmingham, when told of the
strange happening, wondered if the spirits of men who had been
killed around Mons rose to help their comrades.

Stories like the Angels of Mons abounded at that time. Just as
incredible was the tale about the million men of the Russian Army
Corps that landed in Aberdeen on their way to join the BEF in France.
The teller always knew someone who had seen them. The more imaginative among them spiced their tales with the detail of the Russians
even having 'snow on their boots'.

The reality of Mons, though, was plain enough for nurses to see.
Hospital trains loaded with wounded were pouring westwards to
hospitals that were themselves on the move. Sister Luard, who
dressed wounds on the train, told how men had often been lying on

straw in horseboxes for days without toilet facilities. Many of them had gangrenous wounds. Men needing urgent amputations were put off the train on to stretchers on the platform. Nurses were not to attempt anything but swabbing with lysol and then gauze dipped in iodine. Never had Sister Luard seen any wounds like those shrapnel-shell wounds – 'more ghastly than any I had seen or smelt in South Africa'.

One nurse, Jean Wrea, who received them on the platform recalled: 'A very young Second Lieutenant had been lying for two days with an undressed wound in his leg. As soon as I looked at his body I knew it was gangrene. I fetched the surgeon. His examination was quick and decisive. He walked away saying quietly, "The gas has reached his abdomen. There's nothing to be done." I went to look at the others being offloaded.'

The war for those nursing sisters had suddenly changed from an exciting adventure into a frightening reality. What was happening to the British army? Unit war diaries told of battalions marching 200 miles to the rear in thirteen days.

The matron and forty-two nursing sisters of the 9th British Military Hospital joined the general retreat on 26 August. All men on lines-of-communication duties and personnel not needed for front-line battalions were packed at speed into old-fashioned French goods trains. Why? Because the formidable German army of more than four million fully trained soldiers, with overwhelmingly heavy artillery, had broken through French and British lines into Brussels and by 2 September Von Kluck's army was threatening to take Paris.

French troops from the Paris garrison came out in taxi cabs to reinforce the defences. From the metropolis, too, came casualty clearing stations. Accompanying a French CCS was an American woman, known to her patients as Miss Mademoiselle.

She described in letters home that what it was like for those young girls arriving in earshot of the guns of the Marne. She worked with a surgeon who believed he could avoid amputation by continual irrigation of a wound as soon as possible. He took out the debris, then put in tubes for drainage of the wound. Into these tubes a dark liquid was pumped every two hours so that the wound was kept in a constant bath of antiseptic. 'We did between 25 and 35 operations everyday.'

This irrigation treatment, devised by Doctors Dakin and Carrel, certainly reduced the onset of sepsis and gas gangrene from bad wounds and amputations. VAD Gwynnedd Lloyd of the 6th General Hospital, Rouen, who woke men up every three hours to inject the hypochlorus acid solution into wounds, found that the men hated it, as it made the wound so cold and painful. Nevertheless the infection would diminish, and limbs and lives were saved.

In their letters home, nurses found that they could not tell parents all they were doing.

> I thought it would sicken them to think of me putting in drains and washing wounds so huge and ghastly as to make one wonder at the endurance of mankind. Another thing I cannot get hardened to is the last agonies of the dying. When my little number 23 flung out his arms last night to say good-bye, he knew he was going. I can tell you it took all my control to finish my last 34 anti-tetanus injections a few minutes later ...

Strangely enough, many nurses, QAs and VADs, looking back on their wartime days, have said that despite all the tragedies, the work was satisfying, because it felt so worthwhile.

The German advance was held on the Marne. They then withdrew to the high ground overlooking the River Aisne, an almost impregnable position. Urgent messages to base hospitals got them ready for the horrific casualties expected from attacks across the river. Soon casualties were arriving at base in their hundreds each day. The McGuire sisters wrote copious notes in their diaries about terrifying wounds they had dressed. But what disturbed many nurses was the grim truth that casualties were simply overwhelming medical facilities, and doctors just did not have the time to treat them all. On such days one doctor would have the unenviable duty of assessing a man's chances of survival. If a man's wounds were definitely life-threatening he would be placed in a special tent, sometimes called the moribund ward, where he would be made as comfortable as possible until he died. Doctors and nurses expended their precious time on those likely to survive.

Nurses had to deal with a horrific variety of wounds. Sometimes bodies were blasted beyond recognition, or even totally disintegrated, leaving hardly enough of a bloody bundle to put in a grave. In contrast some men died without a mark on their bodies, when the blast of shells ruptured capillaries in the lungs and brain.

Terrible also were the wounds caused by clusters of shrapnel that tore jagged holes in the flesh and carried with them fragments of clothing and foreign matter which infected the wound right away. It was bad enough for army nurses with previous experience in the South African wars but for young women of the Voluntary Aid Detachments it was far worse. Some of them had little more than the

Florence Nightingale,
1820–1910

The fifteen-bedroom house, Lea Hurst, Derbyshire, where Florence Nightingale was living when she heard God calling her to his service. Her nursing commitment began here

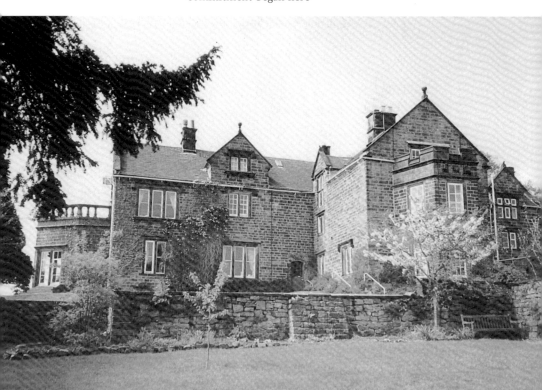

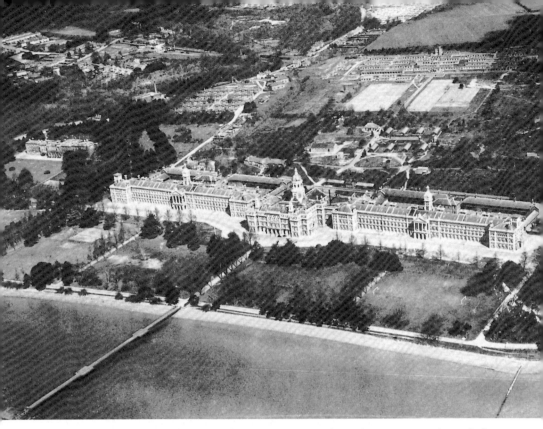

The building of the Royal Victorian Hospital, Netley, was started just before Florence Nightingale returned from the Crimean War. She condemned the plans and suggested alternatives. Despite support from Prime Minister Palmerston, Florence was unable to stop the hospital being built on unsanitary principles with unventilated rooms and all the patients' windows facing north-east, not across the sea. It was completed in 1863 as the chief military hospital in England

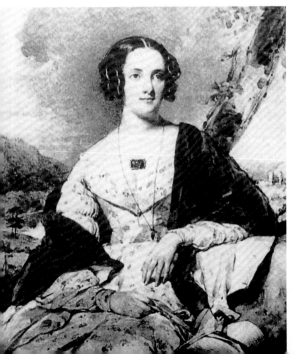

Eliza Mackenzie who organized nurses for the Royal Naval Hospital at Therapia during the Crimean War. As a result, the Royal Navy was pleased to give approval for female nurses in hospitals

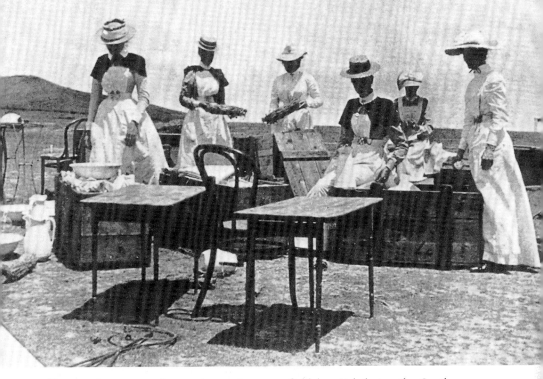

Nursing sisters on active service setting up a field hospital during the South African Boer War (photograph courtesy of the Imperial War Museum, London)

Army nursing sister accompanying a patient to a ward in a mobile field hospital in South Africa (photograph courtesy of the Imperial War Museum, London)

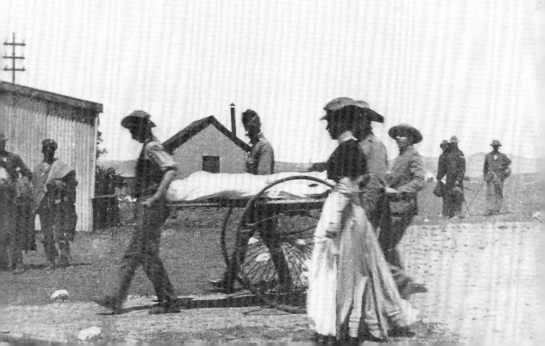

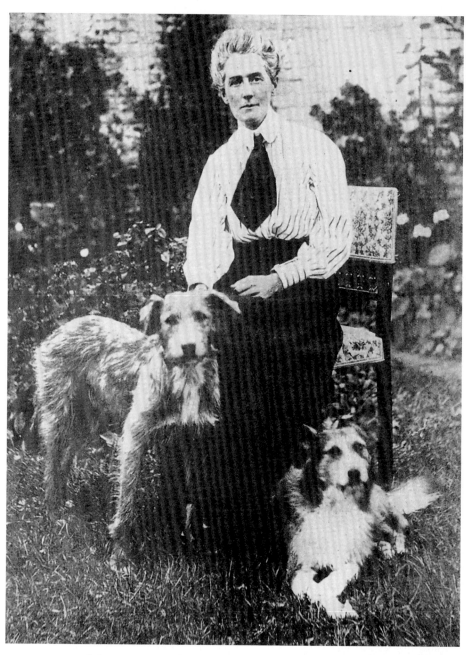

Nurse Edith Cavell, shot by Germans for helping wounded soldiers to escape from advancing German divisions. Her death spurred thousands to enlist

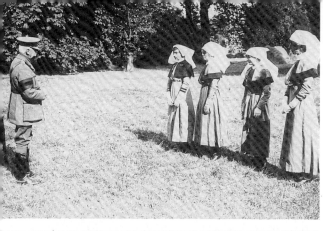

Military medals presented by General Plumer to QAIMNS nursing sisters for gallantry whilst under fire (photograph courtesy of the Imperial War Museum, London)

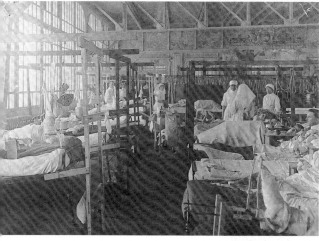

Surgical ward of No. 2 General Hospital, Quai d'Escale, Le Havre. Note the St Clair Thomas fracture beds

Surgical ward, Royal Victorian Hospital, Netley

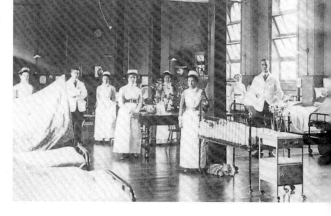

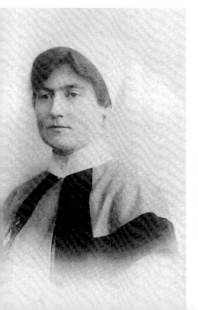

Sister Lilly Grace Petter QAIMNS served in casualty clearing stations in France from 1915 until the war's end in 1918. She often related how, when under canvas near the front-line, she would sleep with an upturned enamel basin protecting her tummy, being fearful of suffering a shrapnel wound there, and aware that she would not be in a position to mind one in the head!

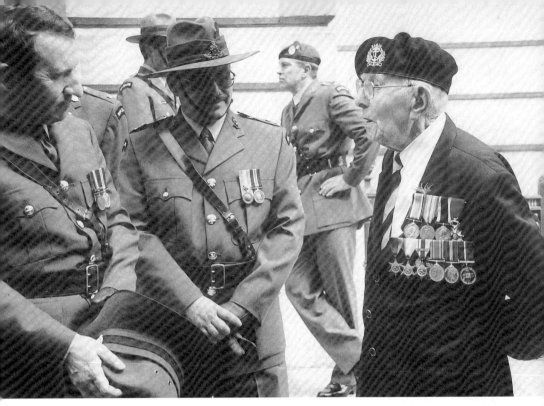

Gallipoli veteran, Fred Bunday, ninety-nine years old, marched to the cenotaph
and stood to attention for half an hour on Anzac Remembrance Day, April 2000

King George V greeting the matron of a casualty clearing station at Remy Sidings,
Ypres, during World War One

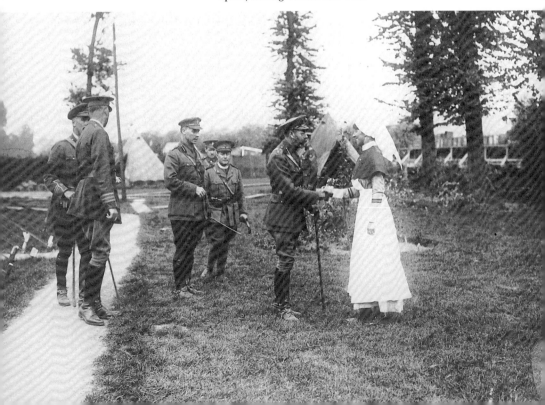

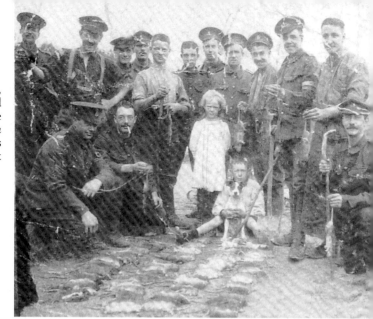

Rats from the trenches, 1916. Sergeant Wilfred Taylor RAMC, the author's father (*first on left, kneeling*) takes time out for a rat hunt

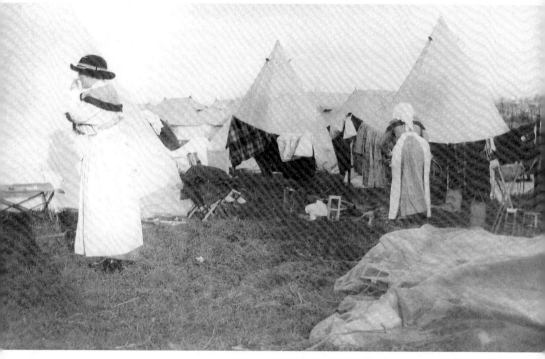

Nursing sisters repairing damage to tents after a storm in France during World War One

Nurses at Huddersfield Infirmary take a break from caring for casualties from France, 1917. (Author's mother *front row, left*)

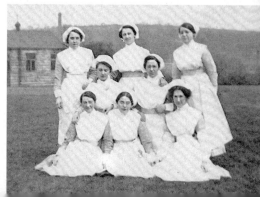

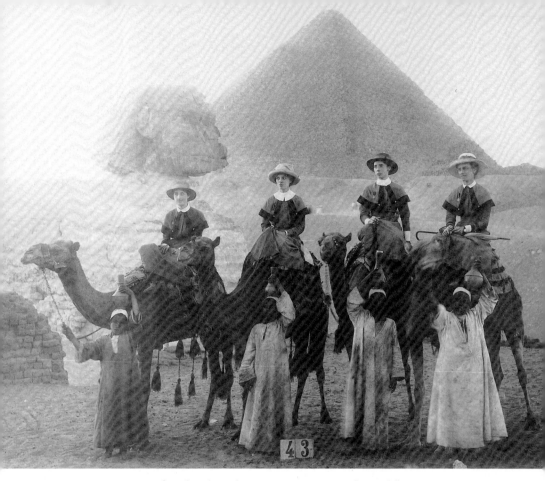

Enjoying a few days leave between campaigns in the Middle East, 1916–17

Soldiers in 1918 did not come home to a land fit for heroes as politicians had glibly promised. Many had to beg, sell bootlaces or matches, sing or make music in the streets. Often returning soldiers, especially those who had been gassed, were too ill to work. Nurses saw the same patients in and out of hospital time after time. Many died prematurely but rarely did their wives receive a pension

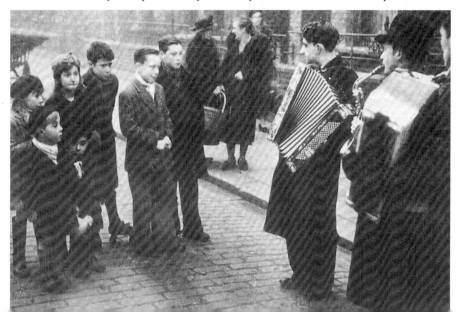

basic training in first aid that a girl guide might have taken, but they were plunged into the thick of the horror. VAD Kathleen Rhodes recalled that doctors 'probed and dressed wounds so terrible that only the most hardened of stomachs could look upon them.'

The flood of casualties brought all the nursing staff much closer together. Experienced QA nursing sisters who once might have kept 'amateur' nurses of the Voluntary Aid Detachments away from serious casualties had them working closely alongside as colleagues. VADs were taking on more responsibilities than matrons at one time would ever have countenanced.

Sister Christina Hastings wrote of a very young soldier who had 'all his genital parts blown off'. It was an awful dressing for her to do every morning. The wound was just a hole with a silver tube coming out of it and the gauze packing the cavity had to be pulled out piece by piece every morning. Sometimes they would give him a drop of brandy afterwards.[6]

Nurses were also coping with casualties far different from any previous wars. Not only were bodies torn apart horrifically by the new killing machines but minds as well. Tremendous advances in weaponry, artillery and explosives had nerve-shattering effects on front-line soldiers.

Charles Moran (later Lord Moran), who served as medical officer to the 1st Battalion of the Royal Fusiliers, wrote of such casualties: 'Men wear out in battle like their clothes. The nerves of the most steadfast of infantrymen can only withstand so much continual shelling and night patrolling especially if they have little rest each day. Add to all that the morale sapping mud, rain, and freezing conditions in a quagmire of trenches and it was not surprising that men's nerves broke.'

News coming into hospitals via soldiers from the front was disheartening and often incredible. Sister Peterkin recorded some in her diary then.

The Middlesex Regiment which left Chatham a thousand strong, just before us, came back past our hospital with fewer than two hundred men.

Soldiers still had on their field dressings and even tourniquets which had not been touched for two days. One young man had both legs off....

A lot of our men were caught in barbed wire entanglements and killed like rats in a trap. A regiment of Hussars was practically wiped out and the 7th General Hospital abandoned 700 beds, tents and equipment in their hurried retreat. Nurses had only what they stood up in.[7]

Nursing sisters in the hospital at Amiens recalled how they got orders to move within ten minutes, taking their wounded with them in cattle trucks. In the 3rd British Military Hospital many of the bed cases were too ill to move, and so four sisters stayed with them when the Germans overran their location.

Sister Peterkin described how she and her colleague often had to pack hurriedly and retreat to a safer area. Sweating and dirty, and packed into a crowded train, they eventually made a slow journey through Le Mans, Nantes and on to Saint-Nazaire, sustained only by one meal of bully beef stew. The role for them now was to take patients to hospital ships sailing between Saint-Nazaire and southern England ports.

Not all men reeling back from the German onslaught were fortunate enough to find a place among those crowded French rail horseboxes. Hundreds of men, often separated from their units, were roaming the countryside trying to make their own way back on foot. In the confusion of that retreat one British nurse became a victim. Her name is legendary.

It happened that some of the walking wounded were lucky enough to reach a small Belgian hospital at Ixelles, which had developed as a school for the training of nurses under the supervision of a well-qualified British nurse, Edith Cavell. She had been in her early forties when she was invited in 1907 to take charge at Ixelles, and for the next seven years had been so successful that the school had earned international renown. It was after the battle of Mons that a trickle of walking wounded from British units, who had been tramping over the countryside evading capture, began to arrive at Ixelles hospital. They had their wounds dressed by Nurse Cavell and another English nurse there, Millicent White (later Bartrum).

By the time soldiers were fit enough for the next stage of the journey back to Britain, the two nurses, helped by the Belgian Resistance, had worked out an escape route through German units to the Dutch frontier. No doubt some of these soldiers had some useful military intelligence – Ixelles was only nine miles away from where the German zeppelins that bombed London were based.

Unfortunately, Edith Cavell and Millicent White innocently believed that those around them were equally committed to helping wounded British soldiers. Security was lax and the German Secret Service exploited existing conflicts between Flemings and Walloons.

This spawned a network of informers ready to give information in return for favourable treatment, or even the return of relatives held as prisoners of war by the Germans.

For months Germans kept the hospital under close supervision. Then, in August 1915, they pounced, arresting Edith Cavell and another English nurse, Elizabeth Wilkins, and throwing them into a damp cell in St Gilles Prison. Unaccountably, Wilkins was soon released, but Cavell was kept in prison on a meagre prison diet for weeks awaiting trial. The court martial began on 7 October. Arraigned with Nurse Cavell before a military court of five German officers were thirty-four members of the French Resistance.

The process was swift and summary. Edith Cavell herself was questioned for only five minutes. During the whole of the hearing she stood perfectly composed and freely admitted to helping wounded British soldiers to escape through Holland.

The next day the prosecutor demanded the death penalty for Nurse Cavell and eight of the others accused. Edith always thought the worst punishment she would get would be imprisonment with hard labour. In any event, she showed no emotion when she was led out of the chamber while the court came to its decision. For three days she waited in her cell. Then at four o'clock on 11 October, the prison governor came into her cell with the verdict. She was to be shot the next morning.

All that night, neutral diplomats made desperate efforts to have the sentence commuted to imprisonment. Cold-blooded German officialdom was unresponsive, however, and determined she should die.

Edith Cavell refused to plead for mercy. She told her chaplain, 'They are going to shoot me simply because Germany hates Britain.'

Early the next morning – the day before her fiftieth birthday – she was taken to the National Rifle Range. There, along with the head of the local Resistance group – the only two of the original thirty-four accused – she was made to stand against a grassy bank and shot.

Nurse Cavell's death was not the end of her story. Days later, newsboys across Britain, howled their headlines: 'Germans shoot Nurse Cavell.' A fury gripped the country. Previous stories of German atrocities – bayonetting French babies, for instance – had largely been dismissed as propaganda. Now the public bayed for blood. Some 40,000 extra recruits joined the army that week. Men and women throughout the land were more resolved than ever to beat the barbaric enemy.

Meanwhile the situation on the Western Front was only too evident in the wards of hospitals and casualty clearing stations, as battle lines moved forwards and backwards. Nurses on makeshift hospital trains risked their lives in many ways during those early months of the war, for in order to get from one carriage to the next without waiting for the train to stop, they often took the hazardous route of clambering along the footboards from one coach to the next. Their lives were also at risk from attacks by German aircraft and shellfire. It was not unusual for hospital trains to arrive at base with windows and roofs shattered.

Shortly after the first battle of Ypres, in October 1914, the 7th Hospital train was standing in the town's railway station with nurses attending to the wounded, when it came under heavy artillery bombardment. Shrapnel killed and wounded orderlies and soldiers helping with the casualties on the train and in the square outside the station. Unfortunately the carriages could not be moved as the engine had gone to Hazebrouk for its water-tank to be refilled. Whilst high explosives rained down upon the station, nurses carried on with their duties.

The battle of Ypres ended in a stalemate of trench warfare. Both Allied and German armies dug themselves deep into a network of trenches on either side of a stretch of no-man's land that ran from the North Sea to the Swiss frontier. Soon those trenches became rat-infested and a health hazard. Sometimes during a quiet spell a rat hunt was organized. Sergeant Wilfred Taylor of the RAMC remembered the way rats were flushed out and killed in the trenches where men fought, ate and fitfully slept during that long period of stalemate.

Military hospitals and casualty clearing stations moved closer to the front lines to ease the evacuation of wounded. Casualty clearing stations were rarely free from enemy shelling and therefore nurses had to be ready at a moment's notice to evacuate personnel or risk further injuries.

Quiet times along the Western Front gave a deceptive impression. Along the 120 miles of trenches a continuous stream of casualties came from sniping, night-time fighting patrols and raids on enemy trenches to capture prisoners for interrogation. Battalion commanders were also keen to show their brigade commanders that they were pursuing the war 'energetically'. There was a mistaken notion in high command that offensive action bolstered the uncertain morale of troops – morale that was beginning to concern commanders ensconced in their comfortable châteaux. Consequently, at regular intervals men were killed and wounded on 'morale-boosting' raids.

Added to wounds inflicted by the enemy were those from the

harsh winter of 1914-15, when even the duckboards of the trenches were under muddy slush. Soldiers were forced to stand in mud up to their knees for days on end. No matter how they tried to dry and warm their feet, many soldiers went back to hospital with painfully swollen 'trench feet', which took months to heal.

For nurses, that first year of the war was more harrowing than any of them could have imagined. Sister Elsie Grey, a New Zealand nurse in her late twenties, told how upset she was: 'Dozens and dozens of boys from the front with an arm or leg off, some even with both arms and legs off. Basket cases. It was awful too, seeing nurses so tired they were collapsing on the floor. Some fast asleep, their heads on kitbags.'[8]

For everyone it was a year of revelation – and seen by many as a year of mismanagement and confusion. Not surprisingly, perhaps, December 1914 ended with a situation (the Christmas Truce) that has been debated ever since.

# 6 Unusually Quiet on the Western Front

'Here shall he see
No enemy
But winter and rough weather.'
William Shakespeare, *As You Like It*, Act II, Sc. 4

On Christmas Eve 1914, while nurses behind the Allied lines in France were preparing for carol singing in the wards, the bleary-eyed men of the Garhwal Rifles were making their way to the front line for a never-to-be-forgotten Christmas.

They shivered in their wet greatcoats as they began the 'Stand to' at dusk in the sour pervasive stench of death. Their nostrils had never got used to that smell throughout those months of unavailing attempts to pierce the German lines. Its impact never diminished. Occasionally a few yards of ground changed hands, frequently at a cost of far too many comrades killed.

Now, on Christmas Eve itself, the Garhwal Rifles were to keep watch on the movements, if any, of the enemy across the hundred yards or so of the shell-pocked mud of no-man's-land. They were not expecting any. For days there had been little sign of life above the parapets on either side, no troops to be seen and only a rare rifle shot heard. Between the two enemies on the water-logged land lay the decomposing bodies of the dead from attacks and counter-attacks.

The Garhwal riflemen trudged to their posts with mud sucking at their boots, weighed down by sodden greatcoats clinging icily to their bodies. With one company was Captain W.G.S. Kenny, buoyed that evening by the thought of the home leave he had been promised, as soon as Christmas was over. Then he would see his baby son, born after he had left for France.

70

Later on, some of his company were slumped on the rough-hewn firestep whilst others kept a look-out. Some smoked surreptitiously, holding their hands cupped around the glowing tip of cigarettes. Many just sat with their head in their hands.

Kenny moved slowly along the line. His legs moved stiffly like those of a mechanical toy. When he reached the end of his company's part of the trench, he peered carefully over the parapet into the night. Occasionally from further down the line, flares rose, illuminating the great loops of barbed wire. What on earth were they all doing here?

A figure sidled up alongside him, Platoon Sergeant Francis.

Suddenly, at precisely 2300 hours, a chorus of voices burst from the German trenches. A volley of rifle fire and shouts merged into a raucous singing of carols. Germans were climbing out of their trench. They stood with arms held high, some carrying bottles. Jovially, slowly they began to walk towards the British lines. Tommies, catching the Christmas spirit, set off to meet them, carrying packets of Woodbines that had come up as presents with the mail that morning.

Kenny and Francis watched, amazed at what they were seeing. Spontaneously German and British soldiers were swopping gifts, fraternizing in the mud by the barbed wire.

From first light the next morning the same spirit of truce and goodwill prevailed. More gifts had come up with the post for the Germans and for the British, too, along with army rations. Every soldier received a present from Princess Mary of a tin box full of cigarettes or pipe tobacco. Non-smokers had chocolate instead and comforts of other kinds galore.

Once again it was a time for British and Bavarian troops to exchange gifts of beer for schnapps and German sausage for plum puddings. A sergeant from the North Staffs appeared dressed like a comic pantomime dame, wearing a woman's skirt and blouse with an umbrella and a top hat that he had found in a nearby ruined house. A huge German gallantly took the dame's hand and danced round and round polka fashion to appreciative applause from Germans and British alike.

Whilst combatants consorted happily, burial parties recovered bodies from water-logged shell-holes, engineers repaired barbed wire and shored up slithering mud-filled sandbags on parapets. Unofficially the truce spread down the line. Nurses heard about it from drivers of ration trucks and ambulances. Sister Muriel Castledine heard the news from am ambulance driver: 'He said the Germans were just ordinary chaps like our own and didn't want to fight anymore than our lads did. We began to hope that the war might yet be over by

Christmas as everyone once believed. It was like a load being lifted off our backs, that life might just get back to normal after all.'[1]

But when the news got back to the commander-in-chief of the BEF, Field Marshal Sir John French, his fury knew no bounds. Signals flew to every unit. This was not a way to win a war. All officers who had taken part were reprimanded and punished. Captain Kenny, who had served with his company gallantly from the very beginning of the campaign, had his leave stopped. Fraternizing in an unofficial truce was unforgivable. Nurses who heard about it still clung to the hope that a sensible peace might come in its wake, but brigade commanders and staff officers, not wanting to lose a safe billet by appearing to condone the fraternization, despatched blistering reprimands to all officers within their command. Such lapses of indiscipline, they averred, were 'totally against the development of the offensive spirit so essential for the winning of the war'. Commanders condoning fraternization would be replaced.

Nevertheless, at eleven o'clock a few nights later, on 31 December, a volley of rapid fire came from the German trenches. Not a bullet came near men on the British side. Realization then dawned. Eleven o'clock in Britain was twelve o'clock in Berlin. German soldiers were celebrating New Year. An hour later, Tommies returned the compliment.

So ended that year of blundering and butchery. The General Officer Commanding was just as determined as his British counterparts that such fraternization would never again occur. It could bring peace and that would never do. An end to promotion and glory.

He prepared an edict ready for the next Christmas. He sent it to all commanders of corps, divisions and brigades. There was to be no repetition of the unauthorized truce. To make sure of this he added: 'the artillery will maintain a slow gun fire on the enemy's trenches commencing at dawn, and every opportunity will be taken to inflict casualties upon any of the enemy exposing themselves.'

For the record it must be mentioned that the truce of December 1914 did in fact linger in the line south of Neuve Chapelle village, until a major offensive was deliberately launched from there against the German positions on 10 March 1915.

Nurses were appalled by the numbers of wounded brought in by stretcher-bearers. Captain Kenny's company with the 1/39th Garhwalis were victims of that slaughter. They advanced in open order, stepping on to lines of bodies of those who had been killed earlier, still in line. Captain Kenny's body was trampled into the mud by the next wave of attacking infantry. He never did hold the baby son he had looked forward to seeing for the first time.

One nurse helping the wounded on to a hospital train recalled a tragic accident: 'One poor man of the Royal Sussex, while helping with some of the wounded this morning, slipped on the rails and had both legs cut off by a passing train. He died two hours afterwards.'[2]

Nursing sisters evacuating wounded on those cattle trucks wondered if that battle for Neuve Chapelle really was vastly more costly for the Germans, as reports from Sir John French made out. In the hospital wards nurses saw the 'victorious offensive' for what it was: a series of savage encounters for an inconsequential gain of ground. It was only too clear to them that hospitals were in grave danger of being inundated with too many casualties for them to treat. Wounded men were being put to bed in the same blood-soaked clothes in which they arrived, until nurses had time to cut off boots and clothing to wash and dress the wounds.

It was at such times that Maud McCarthy, matron-in-chief to the British armies in France, showed her organizing skill, cutting red tape to bring out nursing reinforcements, medical stores and equipment. Daughter of a lawyer, she had passed through the Army Nursing Reserve during the Boer War into the new QAIMNS. Unlike her predecessor at Scutari, the legendary Florence Nightingale, she was a great diplomat, well liked by medical officers of all ranks and by the nurses themselves, as well as being a great administrator. Her work was recognized later in the war when she was made a dame.

Her task in the early days demanded ingenuity when resources were strained to the utmost, as seriously wounded men were brought back by trains and barges to ports in northern France. From there hospital ships waited to take them back to Britain.

Sister Sarah Huggett remembered seeing patients waiting in a dockside warehouse at Boulogne:

I stared horror struck at the scene which met my eyes when I went on duty one evening. Embarkation had started; men on crutches, blind men with eyes bandaged, clung to the shoulder of the man in front in one long column; their clothes were clogged with mud and dried blood; they stumbled over figures lying either dead or asleep on the floor of the huge warehouse; some were actually crawling on hands and knees in case they got left behind. Finally there came the stretcher bearers with the badly wounded, their grey expressionless faces fallen in and hollow cheeked. The miserable procession brought from the slimy black mire of no man's land seemed endless.[3]

Maud McCarthy soon made a difference to that awful scene. With more nurses and medical orderlies brought from Britain, she eased the suffering of those who had lain in pain so long and hastened their return home. There in villages and towns nationwide, through which military hospital trains passed, walls and buildings were plastered with recruiting posters urging young men and women to join one of the services.

Alice Proctor (later Remington) volunteered with the VADs. She saw it as an opportunity for real war service, as did many women from sheltered middle-class homes who realized they were not bound to live a wholly domestic existence. Indeed, they volunteered in their thousands. Some went into the First Aid Nursing Yeomanry, which had been active in France from the opening months of the war, and others for VAD service, which eventually supplied 23,000 nurses and 18,000 orderlies. Regardless of experience, they were flung into hospitals working long hours, often with inadequate facilities.

Alice recalled that she received simple instruction in first aid during which time she learnt the technique of supporting a fractured leg with a couple of broomsticks and some straps, how to stop excessive bleeding with a tourniquet and some rather unorthodox treatment for burns.[4]

Alice Proctor, along with VAD drivers of the motor ambulance unit, was sent to live in a barn at Etaples, and for the next two years slept on a palliasse filled with straw, with layers of newspaper above and below it in an attempt to keep warm.

It was Alice Proctor's job to drive one of the cumbersome Buick ambulances to the local railway station to take wounded off the trains to the hospitals. On a cold morning, starting those old Buicks with a cranking handle demanded a degree of strength not all of them possessed. And if the engine backfired and a nurse had her thumb round the starting handle, it could dislocate or break it.

Trains came in at all hours. In the middle of the night, drivers would be wakened by a shrill whistle and then it was a race for the vehicles.

At the station medical orderlies were responsible for lifting the stretchers into the ambulances but sometimes when they were desperately short of men, those of us who were moderately strong used to help. I always used to go the far end of my ambulance and as orderlies were pushing the stretchers in I would try to stop them from hitting the far end and giving the patient a jolt. Those orderlies were sometimes so tired, that it was a case of, "oh let's get rid of this lot, whoop", like that! Well, if you are badly wounded ...

Some men had dysentery, poor things, that was really terrible because they couldn't be looked after and they were in a shocking state. They were so ashamed of themselves that we girls were cleaning them up and they couldn't help it.

It was very hard for those young girls, most of whom had come from very good homes and had never seen the rougher side of life before joining the VAD. Alice Proctor remembered how one girl was so unnerved by the strain of it all that she threw herself off a cliff to end it all. This might seem hard to believe, but even experienced medical officers could be driven to desperate measures by the stress of seeing so much human suffering. In a hospital off the beaches of Normandy in the Second World War a medical officer slashed his brachial artery and shot himself for the same reason as the VAD girl committed suicide.[5]

Another stressful duty for those young women drivers was burying the dead. After a 'big push' there were often not enough coffins and so the VADs would go to the mortuary and carry the dead in blankets, named and numbered, with those who had been dead longest taken first. They went to the military cemetery and Alice would stand by the padre at the graveside, 'because there was no other woman there for those chaps'.

At the time, Alice, like so many of her colleagues, on those rare occasions when she had home leave, never discussed with her parents the gruesome details of her life overseas. People at home could not really imagine the horror of it all. According to the newspapers, the war had settled into an impasse of trench warfare with occasional costly offensives. Nurses saw the situation as it really was, with a steady stream of wounded coming back to hospitals, even at times when newspaper reports said: 'All quiet on the Western Front'.

It was never so quiet. The Germany quickly adapted their weapons and tactics to the new situation. Siege howitzers lobbed massive shells into British trenches, trench mortars lobbed high-explosive bombs so that they landed almost vertically in the trench itself.

Both sides had to eat, though. So as each day ended, a tacit short truce prevailed in the hinterlands of German and Allied trenches. Limbered horse-drawn waggons rumbled over the cobbled approach roads bringing up rations and ammunition. And under the same cloak of darkness, small parties went out from both sides to collect and bury the dead. Many had already sunk into the fetid, churned-up mud to decompose into a putrescent mass. Medical officer Captain Charles Huxtable RAMC recalled the first day he joined his unit in the front line. That night he went out into no man's land with stretcher parties to pick up any wounded they could find. 'It was a desperately sad sight,' he wrote, 'I can still see in my mind's eye the terrible losses sustained by the Highlanders – bodies lying about everywhere, just as they had fallen.'[6]

Somehow transportation of casualties became less fraught, as a kind of mutual understanding developed between the German and Allied high command. In the quietness of dusk supply roads were not shelled, and ambulances and carts could bring back the wounded on regular runs. Nurses in the base hospitals gradually began to receive casualties in a more orderly manner.

In the early months of 1915 some British doctors and nurses were helping soldiers to recover from amputations by using a new method of blood transfusion developed by Americans of the Harvard Unit and brought to the hospital at Dannes-Camiers. It was a technique that used a solution of sodium citrate to stop the blood from clotting during transfusion. Such transfusions saved the lives of many seriously wounded men who otherwise would have died through excessive loss of blood.

To the hospitals further away from the front wounded soldiers had a smoother though longer passage back, travelling by barge on the canals that ran from casualty clearing stations. Some came too by hospital train.

A steady flow arrived each day. Never did the hospitals have time to clear their beds. They had clearly learnt little from previous abortive offensives. High command initiated experimental offensives to give officers the necessary experience for the much vaunted victorious 'big push'. Inevitably these charges resulted in enormous numbers of casualties pouring into field and base hospitals.

Another serious factor governing nursing services at this time was the extent to which the morale of front-line soldiers was affected by the plight of wounded on the battlefield. They knew how stretcher-bearers often could not immediately get wounded back from where they had fallen. A wounded man might wait for 24 hours or longer before he could be brought back to the rear. Rarely, however, was this due to the stretcher-bearers' lack of courage. Officers often had to make difficult decisions and forbid them to go out when the battleground was under shell and machine-gun fire. In the early days of trench warfare, the wounded were looked after by RAMC stretcher-bearers assisted by regimental aid men. Later, though, two platoons of infantry were seconded to each battalion to act as stretcher-bearers during attacks. So terrible were the muddy conditions that it often took six or eight men up to four hours to carry stretcher cases shoulder high to a casualty clearing station.

The turnover of infantrymen in some battalions was so rapid that subalterns were killed before they had time to learn the names of men in their platoon. Men always knew when another 'big offensive' was near. Drivers of ration trucks told them of piles of ammunition and of wooden crosses partially covered by tarpaulin offloaded in villages behind the line.

Sister Mayne recalled all those terribly wounded men brought back to her hospital after the attempt to break the German lines at Loos in September 1915. Six British divisions attacked for three weeks through the mining villages until the offensive petered out and another 50,000 casualties filled the hospital wards. Nurses had to watch so many of them die.

'There were so many of them, so suddenly and they did not want to die,' recalled Sister Mayne. 'It was an experience which upset us all in various ways for a long time. In our training it was a subject never dealt with. When you have looked after someone for days at a time and you know he's going to die, you just have to put up some kind of defensive wall around your emotions and not show your feelings to patients.'[7]

Early one morning Sister Peterkin and her colleagues were called into the matron's office one at a time. With the hospital matron sat the visiting principal matron. She asked Sister Peterkin if she had any complaints. Was there anything she would like to see changed in the hospital? Had she written any letters home or to nursing journals complaining of conditions?[8]

Apparently a nurse had written to one of the nursing journals describing the inadequate conditions in her hospital and had got some of her colleagues to sign the letter. The censor had stopped it. The principal matron wanted to make sure no one else had similar ideas and so she was seeing every nurse to find out if there were any genuine complaints. The nurse who had written the letter was posted to Le Havre.

Three months later, Sister Peterkin was herself posted to a duty she had never imagined herself performing. She was to be sister-in-charge of two hospital barges! There were five flotillas, each comprising six barges. They travelled in pairs towed by steam tugs and floated patients more or less in peace and comfort along certain French and Belgian canals from advanced casualty clearing stations to base hospitals.

Each pair of barges was commanded by an RAMC medical officer with the rank of captain, and on each barge was one nursing sister, one staff nurse, an RAMC sergeant, corporal, three nursing orderlies, two general duties orderlies, a cook and a cook's assistant. In charge of the navigation was a sergeant of the Royal Engineers and two sappers of the Inland Water Transport Branch.

For these flotillas, the government had requisitioned huge coal barges. They were painted grey on the outside and a bright cream colour inside with white cupboards. Surprisingly the barge could accommodate thirty beds, each with a bedside locker. A hand lift was available for loading and unloading patients where necessary. All barges were equipped with electric light.

It was an 'eye opener' for Sister Peterkin when she first went aboard as she wrote in her diary:

Outside was painted a large Red Cross and there were also red and white striped awnings for when the hatches were off. The top decks were curved but around the outside was a very narrow flat ledge on which it was possible to walk from one end of the barge to the other. There was no hand-rail and only a wooden edge, half an inch high. We all felt nervous walking along this ledge as there was quite a steep drop into cold dirty water for anyone who tripped. In frosty weather it was particularly hazardous to walk along this ledge. More than once in icy weather, I was reduced to crawling ignominiously on my hands and knees to avoid falling into the frozen canal.

Sometimes a barge would take a full load comprising 3,000 of the walking wounded. An RAMC Sergeant and Corporal allocated places on benches to patients according to the severity of their wounds. The doctor and nurse then came round dealing with serious injuries first. Following the doctor and nurse were trained medical orderlies who carried out simple treatment and dressings. After all casualties had been seen, men were seated at a table for a hot meal and a mug of tea.

I usually had bed patients to look after and when their wounds had been dressed I went round hurriedly taking details for diet sheets, and taking temperatures and pulses. The barges travelled so smoothly, patients never noticed the movement.

Sometimes we took patients almost straight from the firing line, or, if there was much fighting going on nearby, with a corresponding rush of patients in the CCS we had them passed straight on to us in an unwashed condition. Our first job then was to dress the wounds, wash all patients and get them into clean pyjamas. This was necessary as the men were nearly always verminous.

We travelled only in daylight and so in winter, with short days we did not travel very far. One reason for travelling only by daylight was having to pass under bridges which sometimes gave us barely an inch of clearance at each side.

We had no time for rest. Even when we had delivered the patients we had to scrub out the barge, inspect all medicine cupboards and re-stock them where necessary. Whilst this was going on, the Nursing Sister would be given a little time off to slip into the nearest village to buy fresh fruit and vegetables for the crew and patients.

Although each barge was fitted with electric lights, no lights were allowed at night time, in case we were attacked by German aeroplanes. This meant we had to juggle with a carefully guarded torch and as we went round the beds at night. Often we sat in inky blackness meditating on the number of patients who might be liable to hemorrhage at any moment.

Night duty on those barges was an unenviable task but it was as nothing compared with the new horror which the German army unleashed on the soldiers who were carried to our barges late in the summer of 1915.

# 7 A Problem for Nurses

'It was a most distressing experience for the doctors and nurses in the hospitals to witness men writhing in agonies which they could do little or nothing to alleviate.'[1]

General Sir John Hay Beith, CBE, MC

A new kind of warfare began on the warm, sunny Thursday of 22 April 1915. Two French divisions were defending a part of the line near the Yser canal to the north-east of Ypres. At four in the afternoon, German artillery bombarded the whole area – trenches and villages alike – for ninety minutes and then suddenly stopped. All was quiet as forward French and Algerian infantry rose carefully in their trenches to look anxiously over no man's land for attacking German infantry.

What they saw puzzled them. They called their officers to come and look for themselves. A strange, greenish-yellow cloud was rolling slowly towards them. What on earth could it be? Then like a thick early morning mist it enveloped men in the trenches. They gasped in agony, noses and throats burning as though scorched; others collapsed and suffocated to death. A cloud of chlorine gas, three times heavier than air, had been released from cylinders in the German trenches. It billowed across no man's land on a light breeze and rolled into the French trenches.

Soldiers ran blindly behind their lines in crazy circles, screaming in agony and clutching their throats. Canadians to their flanks looked on uncomprehendingly, but only for a few moments as they moved to cover the gap in the line against German infantry now advancing. Then the Germans stopped on orders, waiting for the gas to disperse.

When the wounded poured into casualty clearing stations, doctors and nurses strove desperately to help the victims of this gas attack. They had nothing to relieve the soldiers' agony.

Afterwards, on learning more about this grisly new development, medical staff wondered why Allied high command had persistently ignored the warnings it had been given about German plans to use gas warfare. German prisoners under interrogation had freely told of gas cylinders being brought into front-line trenches; a German deserter had described tubes of choking gas placed in batteries of twenty every 40 metres along the front; and a Belgian spy actually pinpointed the location of these lethal tubes. A French spy, Charles Lucieto, had even watched a German demonstration of the gas before Kaiser Wilhelm and senior government and military officials.

He told of how a military band had played martial music to entertain observers while the somewhat reluctant victims of the attack – a flock of sheep a mile away – were gathered in the corner of a field. A naval gun fired the gas shells, which landed reasonably close to the sheep. No explosion followed the landing of each shell, but a greenish-yellow cloud drifted towards the livestock, covering them like a mountain mist. When it had moved over and away from the sheep not one of them moved. They were all dead, and the Kaiser and his ministers drove away.

Though all this information passed into the files of Allied military intelligence, only half-hearted efforts were made to provide protection for soldiers – soldiers who soon would take the place of those sheep.

The possibility of a German attack preceded by poisonous gas was only given serious consideration when Germany accused Britain of shelling German trenches with an asphyxiating gas. The idea behind the German accusation was to make it look as though Germany were retaliating rather than initiating the use of gas warfare. Even so, the Allies took little notice of that broadcast. They were far too preoccupied with their own plans to solve the stalemate in the trenches.

Something new had to be tried.

While the British experimented in secret with prototypes of a tank that could move over the mud-filled, shell holes of no man's land, the Germans were busy developing their own secret weapon – gas.

So it was that before the Second Battle of Ypres began, the Allies had made only a few half-hearted efforts to provide soldiers with some form of protection against gas.

Improvised gas masks were made from pads of cotton-wool held together by gauze and sprinkled with caustic soda provided in beer bottles. These were to be held over nostrils and mouth. The result of those trials was seen in the bottom of trenches that were littered with wool and beer bottles thrown away by men who found they could not breathe at all when those pads were held against the nose and mouth.

Sister K. Luard QAIMNS, in a casualty clearing station a few miles south of Ypres, had first-hand experience of treating a medical officer who had been testing experimental gas masks. He had been using wool soaked in various antidotes to chlorine, but he had inhaled too much chlorine and was choking. He had to be given fumes of ammonia until he could breathe properly again.[2]

Some attempts were made to manufacture a gas helmet made of thick blanket-type flannel in which were sewn mica eye-pieces. The idea was to put the helmet over the head, tuck the flannel under the uniform collar and breathe in through the flannel and out through a tube held in the mouth. The flannel, previously soaked in some foul-smelling liquid, was supposed to neutralize the effects of poisonous gas. Some soldiers had panic attacks, feeling they could not breathe through the foul-smelling flannel.

The resources of medical provision on all fronts were stretched to the extreme, dealing with all the battle casualties from the probing attacks on German positions. Sister C. Mayne took charge of a ward situated in a seminary that had been commandeered as a military hospital. Such was the volume of wounded that sometimes there was a shortage of dressings, nurses were sometimes forced to take drastic measures, improvising bandages from their own 'body linen'.

Sister Mayne wrote in her diary:

> We dealt with the most severe cases first and put them into beds whilst the less severe sat about the floor and around the stove munching rations. Many were asleep as soon as they sprawled upon the floor, others in pain with their wounds still slept without morphia after they had been dressed. We had time for nothing but dressing wounds, administering saline for shock and trying to ease the nightmare of suffering around us.[3]

Tetanus was another dreaded complication, as Elsie Grey recalled.

> There were more tetanus cases coming in too then so we had to be on the go giving tetanus injections as well as the usual run of the mill jobs like removing bits of shrapnel and bullets that did not need the surgeon's skill.

Tetanus was a condition which became an increasingly serious problem which nurses had to cope with as wounded men were brought into hospital after having been lying for hours on the muddy ground of No-Man's Land. The soil there contained spores of the tetanus bacterium which infected wounds and acted on nerve tissues causing muscular spasm. It would be after about ten or more days that a wounded man would begin to complain that his jaw was getting stiff – people talked of it as 'lock jaw' – and then his neck, shoulders and legs would stiffen with painful muscle cramps. In very bad cases, I've heard of men whose muscles got into such an extreme form of spasm that the whole body was arched into a bow so that only the heels and back of the head touched the bed.

The risk of this extreme condition was reduced if tetanus anti-toxin was given as soon as possible after casualties were admitted. It was important but took a lot of time.

Whilst we were in Furnes, shells and bombs dropped every day. One afternoon, a battalion of infantry troops was lined up to be inoculated against typhoid and shells dropped right into the middle of them. We heard a spy must have informed the Germans and someone in charge of the railway station was shot the next morning.

Early one morning the yard outside the seminary was filled with old London buses. We were told to have all patients ready to move as soon as possible as the Germans were pushing through our lines. Then the order was countermanded and the buses drove away. Towards evening that day the place they left in the yard was covered by wounded on stretchers. We stumbled amongst them dressing their wounds, our hands sticky with blood. My legs felt weak and I tottered trying to save myself from falling onto the stretchers. I remember that a verse from childhood then kept running through my mind keeping me going:

> Oh fear not at a time like this
> And thou shalt know ere long
> How sublime a thing it is
> To suffer and be strong!

Serious faced men brought news from the Ypres salient. It was so depressing. There was no hope of getting out of Ypres or holding the salient. But we had to try to keep a cheerful look on our faces. The men responded to what we said. I remember one of them said over and over again as I was dressing a painful wound: "Just keep talking, Sister. Just keep talking."[4]

Mixed with the casualties from high explosive shells were those from gas. After the chlorine shells came the menace of mustard gas. When these new shells landed on Allied positions they belched their fog. They stained the earth where they burst, and when liquid splashed clothing it evaporated and soldiers breathed burning vapour into their lungs. Wherever liquid touched the skin, bulbous blisters arose and if any went into the eye temporary or permanent blindness was assured.

Men who washed and shaved in rainwater taken from shell holes were afflicted too; skin and gums blistered. Men who made tea from apparently clear pools of water by the trenches suffered severe vomiting and pain.

By 27 May when the Second Battle of Ypres ended, Allied losses were appalling. Two miles of muddy land had been lost along with 60,000 British and Commonwealth lives. Nurses never forgot the pathetic state of those casualties packed into their wards, especially the gas patients for whom they could do so little.

'Those casualties were really horrendous,' wrote Elsie Grey. She was a 28-year-old New Zealand nursing sister at 59th British Hospital, when military and civilian gas casualties came into her ward for the first time. 'It was the most horrific sight I've ever seen. Most were blind, and gas had affected the pulmonary tract. Some older French women with the group all died most pathetic deaths. We did not know what to do with them.'

Sister Peterkin had a shocking experience with gas casualties on her evacuation barge.

We took them down into the barge where there was a terrible lack of air for even healthy soldiers to breathe but for the gas victims it was terrifying to see them fighting for breath. Soon after they were loaded, the air coming off their clothing was heavy and stale making their struggle for breath worse. We all felt miserably helpless. What were we to do with them?

Everywhere was so crowded. We had two rows of stretchers slung up on either side of the ward and rows of stretchers resting underneath and wedged close against each other with handles interlocked. The nights were especially bad for the patients had not been undressed and their clothing still exuded the smell of gas. When we did take off their clothes and wash their bodies, we found many of them were covered in huge water blisters. Some had burst and smelt pungently.

It was difficult to keep them alive during the journey back to base. Yet the patients seldom grumbled. They were incredibly cheerful and full of courage.

More than once after evacuating such a load, I've felt quite gassed myself with sore eyes, sickness and raw breathing tubes.[5]

The distress of gas victims was always pitiful for nurses to see. Casualties lay frothing at the mouth or retching and vomiting. Their chests were distended and coughing was so obviously painful. Later thick mucus, copiously dotted with bright red blood, dribbled from the nose and mouth. Blood oozed into tissues of the lungs, which swelled to twice their normal size. Men drowned in their own secretions. It was a horrible death. Neither doctors nor nurses could do much to prevent it.

The accepted treatment nurses gave to casualties can be pieced together from the war diaries some of them kept. The basic method was that nurses should speak to the patient firmly but gently so as to reassure him that he was going to be all right. If in doubt at all about the man's mental condition, they were to treat him for shock as well.

After that, the next priority for nurses was care of a man's eyes. Again he was to be told that blindness was not bound to be permanent even though they looked awful with pus oozing from beneath swollen and painful lids and conjunctivae. Ideally nurses tried to bathe a patient's eyes frequently with sodium bicarbonate, but with a full ward, time was against them.

As months passed, the German army brought out new forms of gas attacks. They stopped discharging gas from cylinders in their own lines because wind-borne gas attacks were too risky for their own troops. A change of wind direction would bring a poisonous gas cloud eddying back into their own lines.

From 1916 onwards both sides were using gas delivered by artillery and mortar shells. Soldiers who saw those strange green clouds approaching panicked. They had seen too many comrades coughing up their lungs before they died. Phosgene gas was colourless, however, and with the rather attractive smell of new-mown hay. It was an asphyxiant, three times heavier than air and ten times more deadly than chlorine. Its effect was horrendous. The gas broke down capillaries, causing mucus to ooze into the lungs so that the patient died of asphyxiation through lack of oxygen. It had a delayed effect upon the heart, too, causing total collapse.

Later, the gas masks issued to troops, though clumsy, did provide protection if used promptly. Therefore it became compulsory for all troops and nurses in front-line areas to carry their gas masks until the war was over.

For doctors and nurses it was the lung-irritant gases that caused the most harrowing of casualties. Day by day, nurses found patients having severe difficulty with their breathing and suffering more intensely. Nurses could clearly see the changes taking place: the face

and neck turning a typical cyanosed blue, the pulse rate rising alarmingly and, unless oxygen was given, the inevitable onset of heart
failure.

Desperately nurses sometimes tried postural drainage to relieve
the 'waterlogging' of the lungs from the patient's exudate. Postural
drainage involved the patient lying face downward with buttocks
raised above chest and the patient was assisted to produce 'paroxysms
of coughing' so that sputum was removed from the lungs. But realis-
tically whatever treatment should have been given was governed by
the time available. Convalescence could be a long and tiresome
process for both nurses and patients. Fresh air and rest were the first
requirements and all strain on the heart and lungs had to be avoided.

As General Sir Douglas Haig clung on to salients at an appalling
cost, into the care of nurses came hundreds of hoarse, blistered,
blinded and vomiting British soldiers. These the poet Lieutenant
Wilfred Owen immortalized before he too was killed: 'Bent double,
like old beggars under sacks, knock-kneed, coughing like hags' until
blood came 'gargling from froth corrupted lungs.'[6]

So effective were gas shells that by the end of the war 125,000
tons of gas were fired at Allied troops. The Allies countered with
their own brands and by 1918 chemical warfare casualties on both
sides exceeded the million mark.

From 1915 onwards, though, casualties of a totally different nature
were coming into hospitals, causing doctors and nurses grave concern.
They were men who, while physically unharmed, were mentally inca-
pacitated by the horror of continuous bombardment and attacks over
the mud and barbed wire of no man's land. For want of a better term
for their diagnosis, medical staff called them 'shell-shock cases'.

George Littlefair, even at the age of 101 remembered vividly what
it was like. With feeling he declared that it would be impossible for
anyone who had never seen a soldier suffering from shell-shock to
understand how it was for those young men.[7]

Regimental medical officers had to treat men who seemed to have
had what they sometimes described as a nervous breakdown. Other
doctors' reports listed the strange symptoms exhibited by such mental
casualties. Patients were shaking hysterically, some were partially
blinded, others could no longer speak, some were deaf, some shivered
in cold sweats, and others were unable to move an arm or leg as if
partially paralysed, despite there being no apparent physical cause.

'Some of these men could hardly do anything for themselves. Even
simple habitual tasks of washing and shaving proved beyond them,'
said George Littlefair.

It was a condition found in all front-line soldiers whatever their nationality. German medical officers had a simple term for it, *Kriegsneurose* – war nerves. French doctors diagnosed it as *la condition mentale de la guerre*.

The problem with which every doctor and nurse had to grappel was how to get such men back into their combat units. Furthermore there was always the question at the back of everyone's mind of how far the mental condition was genuine and how far faked. After all, it was a potentially effective means of getting away from the trenches and on a boat back to Blighty.

The mental stress these men suffered would today be treated by psychiatric therapy, but in those days, the British high command decided to give such casualties a much harsher diagnosis – 'cowardice' – for which men were to be court-martialled. The punishment for the guilty was being shot at dawn by a firing squad drawn from their own regiment. The reasoning behind this harsh policy was that soldiers should fear running away more than they feared the enemy.

Nevertheless, as months of trench warfare went by, 'shell-shock' cases increased alarmingly. Within four months of the opening barrages of the war, medical estimates showed that one officer in ten and one in twenty-five of the other ranks reported sick with some sort of mental breakdown. The depletion of infantry battalions through exhaustion, battle fatigue, hysterical paralysis, or 'shell-shock', for want of a more accurate medical term, alarmed the War Office so much that they sent a specialist consultant neurologist to France to investigate at first hand the strange problems of mental breakdowns in the British Expeditionary Force.

By 1916 articles appearing in national newspapers told of soldiers returning home from France with wounded minds, men who were suffering from 'hysterical blindness', deafness and paralysis. Alarm bells rang louder in the Cabinet. All this publicity was definitely prejudicial to public morale. Politicians and generals feared the spread of anti-war sentiments. Something had to be done. Nurses received a variety of conflicting instructions.

The truth was that no one in government or the War Office was prepared to acknowledge the unsurprising fact that men imprisoned for long periods in mud-filled trenches, bombarded by day and night, and often lying alongside the dismembered bodies of their pals, would sooner or later crack. Those who were lucky were sent back as casualties to the care of nurses in hospitals.

One infantry officer, Siegfried Sassoon – wounded by a bullet in his shoulder during an attack for which he was awarded the Military Cross – described vividly in his diary what life in the trenches was like for those men of his regiment. 'Dead men and living were lying against the side of the trenches – one never knew which were dead and which living. Dead and living were nearly one, for death was in all our hearts.'[8]

Indeed some men were so shattered mentally that they could no longer bear waiting for the inevitable and courted death by exposing themselves unnecessarily in forays into no man's land. They would, for example, run out to bring back a wounded colleague, even when the area was being swept by machine-gun fire. 'Such men were shell-shocked, otherwise they would not have dreamed of doing such a thing,' wrote Sassoon.

Nurses looking after officers suffering from mental breakdown at the National Hospital for the Paralysed and Epileptic in Bloomsbury were often as frightened as the patients by the treatment on offer. For example, Dr Lewis Yealland believed in curing cases of hysteria by administering painful electrical shocks.[9]

The methods employed were far more brutal than the electrical convulsive therapy (ECT) employed in the Second World War, as for example at Number 6 Base Psychiatric Centre, attached to the 95th British General Hospital, Algiers, during the North African campaign. Even there in 1943, it was so frightening that the commanding officer recorded in the unit war diary that the orderlies deserved 'danger money'. It was even more frightening for the patients who told each other what happened when they were strapped down to the bench and electrodes were placed on their foreheads.[10]

But this ECT was mild stuff compared with the drastic, near 'kill or cure' measures sometimes employed by Dr Yealland in 1916. He was determined to show that he could get men to go back to their units more quickly than doctors working at other hospitals.

Various methods were used. The end of a lighted cigarette was touched to the end of a patient's tongue; hot plates burnt the back of his throat when his mouth was kept open by surgical instruments; strong electrical shocks were given to the mouth, neck, and spine. Yealland regarded them all as malingerers. Treatment administered in a locked room became a battle of wills between patient and Yealland.[11]

Nurses heard harrowing tales from patients who came back from some of those extended sessions. But Yealland and others like him justified their methods by the serious nature of the whole problem.

They cited the pressure put on the medical officers by the government to get the men either back to their regiments quickly or discharged into civil life as 'fit' so that they could not claim disability pensions later.

Treatment at other centres was not so cruel. At Craiglockhart, for example, where Siegfried Sassoon spent some time, patients received psychotherapy from Dr William Rivers, formerly a neurologist and anthropologist at Cambridge University. He had tried using psychotherapy to help infantrymen back to their units when he was on the staff of the Red Cross Military Hospital at Maghull, near Liverpool. The hospital had been built in 1912 as a convalescent unit for epileptic patients, but so great was the need for rehabilitation of 'shell-shock' soldiers that the building was requisitioned by the War Office and staffed by army doctors and nurses.

Generally, patients there were confined to their beds and tended sympathetically by nurses unless they became too agitated. This therapeutic period of relaxation, together with analysis of the soldiers' troubles, restored some patients to physical and mental fitness. But others simply could not face a return to front-line service.

The question preoccupying divisional and brigade commanders all the time was how were these men, who had received so little military training, to be kept in the line and made willing to go over the top to attack when ordered? The only solution they could muster between them as motivation was the instilling of fear. A greater fear than the possibility of being wounded or killed. The fear of a quick court-martial and its sentence of death at dawn.

Thus it was that Joseph Byers, who aged sixteen in November 1914 had lied about his age to join a fighting regiment and was on the boat to France on 5 December after only two weeks' training, was hurriedly tried by court martial and shot at dawn. He was just seventeen years old. Members of the court heard from the senior officer that 'We need an extreme example.'

Fusilier Herbert F. Burden, who also had enlisted in 1914, aged sixteen, had fought bravely with the 1st Northumberland Fusiliers for nine months before his mind could take no more and cracked in July 1915. His 'treatment' was a hastily convened court martial for cowardice in which he was found guilty and sentenced to be executed. By whom?

That too was all part of the brutal therapy to cure others who might suffer the same loss of nerve. John Rea Laister, a soldier in young Burden's regiment, recalled how the regimental orderly corporal woke him up before first light one morning and with several others from the Northumberland Fusiliers was marched with loaded rifles to the edge of a wood. They were lined up and watched as young Herbert Burden, escorted by two military policemen was marched across a muddy patch of ground and made to stand with his back to a tree and blindfolded. Laister's squad was then ordered to aim and fire. 'I don't know how they could order that. It was judicial murder,' he said.[12]

The same fate befell former cabin-boy William Hunter, who had served so well with the Loyal North Lancashire Regiment that when he too was court-martialled for cowardice, GOC Henry Wilson was so impressed with the seventeen-year-old's record that he recommended the punishment for his charge of desertion be commuted to prison rather than execution. His recommendation was overruled and young Hunter was shot at dawn. Five boys were among the 306 soldiers shot at dawn.

Men who were mentally disturbed as well as physically wounded were treated in hospitals by more sympathetic nurses. They ensured the men had rest and time to recuperate before they were sent back to be shot at again. Such casualties were kept apart from other wounded soldiers. Care had to be taken not to let other troops know that there was a way out of the line other than feet first.

Major General John Hay Beith recollected visiting a crowded dock-shed in Southampton, where stretchers were packed from end to end with wounded waiting to be taken on to base hospitals. In one corner, kept apart from the rest of the casualties, lay the shell-shock cases. They were being treated by a mesmerist from London, 'called in to lull their wandering, unhappy minds, if he could, into some sort of restful oblivion'.

At that time (1917) London and all the major provincial cities were crowded with troops. Everywhere khaki-clad men were having a last frenzied fling, downing their pints in the pubs, going to theatres and coming out singing martial, patriotic songs put over by ageing baritones and buxom, flag-waving chorus girls. It was as if the people did not really believe in the reality of the war, as if it had for them no great cataclysmic significance when they waved goodbye to their menfolk.

No wonder Lieutenant Owen, back in the front line after being in hospital in Britain, could write so bitterly about the public doing nothing to stop the slaughter. Angrily, Owen wrote what many a nurse surely felt at that time too, that those who could see such pitiful sights,

. . . would not tell with such high zest
To children ardent for some desperate glory.
The old lie: Dulce et decorum est
Pro patria mori.[13]

# 8 Nursing in the Sideshows

'A bloody balls-up.'
Robert Graves, *Goodbye to all that*

Early in 1915 many nurses serving in military hospitals in Britain were surprised to receive posting orders to proceed on embarkation leave. They were not told their destination. But they heard it was not France.

The British War Council believed that because all attempts to break through the German lines on the Western Front had failed, the Allies should try to weaken Germany by campaigns elsewhere, perhaps even forcing an entry into Germany through the east. So it was that within a few months of their embarkation leave, nurses found themselves tending British casualties from campaigns in Turkey, Serbia, Greece, Italy, Mesopotamia, Palestine and East Africa.

On 24 April 1915, 200 ships sailed from Mudros Harbour on the island of Lemnos for the beaches of Gallipoli, on the southwest peninsula of European Turkey. The Allies aimed at putting turkey, Germany's ally, out of the war and opening a sea route to the Black Sea, through which they could supply munitions to their ally, Russia. With Turkey defeated, Britain, France and Russia could attack Germany from the east, through Bulgaria and Romania.

The campaign began in a welter of blood, confusion and amazing courage, which resulted in five Victoria Crosses being won on one beach alone within a few hours of the landing. Casualties were enormous. Nothing went according to plan.

In the early morning mists of that Sunday, 25 April, the first boats carrying British, Australian and New Zealand infantry stealthily approached their beaches. But when they had almost reached land, they milled about in confusion. Half whispered cries were heard. 'We're on the wrong beach, for God's sake! Pull back out.' But the boats behind misinterpreted the confusion and pushed the leading boats further forward, sending in even more troops.

Machine-guns opened fire, raking the whole area. To the horror of their commanders, instead of landing on a beach with gentle slopes leading to the high ground beyond, they had been left on a narrow strip of shore, hemmed in by steep hills and covered by thorny scrub. Men tried to climb precipitous slopes while heavy fire came down upon them from above. Officers lost touch with men and units became hopelessly mixed up and lost.

From that navigational error, one catastrophic blunder followed another. Two thousand men packed into an old collier converted into a kind of infantry landing-craft leapt into water chest high. Many were drowned as the weight of equipment pulled them under, or were mown down by Turkish artillery and machine-gun fire as they waded ashore.

Further advances from any of the beaches were impossible.

Stretcher-bearers staggered down the scrub-covered cliffs in an endless stream, carrying casualties on to the beach. There the wounded lay waiting to be taken by barges that were running an essential shuttle service to hospital ships anchored off shore. While wounded lay on the beach they were under fire from Turks who over-looked the area from three sides. Everyone – from generals to privates – was under fire. Off shore, on the hospital ships, the nurses were often under shell-fire too as they helped to load the wounded from the small boats.

The foothold on the beach was so cramped that there was no room for hospital facilities even of the most primitive kind. Consequently nurses had to make trips in lighters to bring casualties to hospital ships, anchored close to the shore.

The Turks, surprised by the landing of so many troops in such a small area, dug a line of trenches to confine British troops to the tip of the peninsula. Their barbed wire was hung with the corpses of men who had tried to cut a way through. The numbers of wounded grew almost impossible for medics to cope with. The Australian Medical Corps had had two men killed, four missing and eighteen wounded on the first day. Those who were left tended wounded on the beaches under conditions of appalling difficulty while fragments of shell and shingle from bursts of high explosives flew around them and their dressing stations.

Out of a total of 2,500 casualties, over 1,700 wounded were evacuated to hospital ships on that first day.

Sister Mary Brown with her colleagues of the QAIMNS were then serving on the hospital ship *Devanha*, anchored just off Anzac Cove. Shells were whistling overhead and machine-gun bullets from Turkish positions on the cliff-top caves cracking around them. They helped sick and wounded on board from lighters and small boats plying to and from the shore.

Weeks went by, and it became apparent to opposing commanders all along the front that while the Anzac soldiers could not be pushed off the beaches nor could they advance. Four months later, in an attempt to break the deadlock, the British attempted another landing further up the peninsula at Suvla Bay. The landing was unopposed but instead of making for the high ground immediately, battalions brewed tea, formed up and slowly moved towards the hills overlooking the beach. Among them was the 32nd Field Ambulance of the RAMC. Stretcher-bearers attempted to bring in wounded while the main force withdrew. Seventeen of these stretcher-bearers disappeared completely. Their loss was all the more lamentable because four of those seventeen were brothers. They were never heard of again and their bodies were never found.

With the Suvla Bay landings the assault troops failed to reach their objectives. Incompetent generals did not try again.

As the campaign dragged on, nurses were dead-tired, but there was no end to the wounded being carried down to the sea shore. Some men had eaten nothing for days and had had no proper sleep for weeks. Despite the display of red crosses, hospital ships and medical personnel were continually at risk from land-based artillery units, and mines sown on approaches to the beaches.

It was difficult for all those nurses to avoid showing in their faces the shock of seeing a boatload of shattered humanity, as fierce battles raged along the beach area. 'It was a continual boom and crack,' Sister Brown recalled in a letter home. Turks fired shells and machine-guns from the shore and British battleships kept up continual fire alongside them. So busy were the nurses, recalled Mary Brown, that they dressed nearly a thousand wounded one morning and 'were hard at it all day', before sailing for the military hospital on the green island of Lemnos at dawn the following day.[1]

The Australian and British base hospitals on the island eventually had beds for 9,000 casualties. Base hospitals in Cairo, Malta, Alexandria, Gibraltar and Britain took patients fit to travel by sea.

Nurses on RMS *Aragon* often had to cope with twice as many patients as the ship had been designed to accommodate. It was the same with the hospital ship *Gloucester Castle*. On one very bad day, 400 extra wounded men were taken on board and had to lie on mattresses placed side by side on the open deck. Whenever practical, the most seriously wounded men were placed close to the operating theatre, where the surgeon and his team of nurses got to work as soon as the first one arrived. After the operation, casualties were taken down to the ship's wards. Hospital ships often had to stop to hold a brief committal service before sliding over the ship's side the bodies of soldiers who had died of wounds.

Throughout those sea journeys of nearly a hundred miles to Mudros, nurses had always to be ready for the eventuality of the ships being mined. Then they would have to put into practice the drill for saving as many patients as possible in the short time available. On one journey nurses saw a high pillar of smoke and flames shoot up from the deck of the battleship *Bouvet*. She steamed on for a short way and then suddenly, still steaming, capsized and slipped to the bottom with her captain and 623 sailors.

In those overcrowded hospital ships facilities were absolutely appalling. Dysentery cases lay in the fetid air below decks amid the filth from previous cargoes, while those with suppurating or gangrenous wounds were carried on deck. A bedpan was a luxury hardly ever seen. It takes little imagination to visualize what those hospital ships looked like once they reached a port after five days on voyage. Apart from lying in their own excrement men were dehydrated, emaciated and dying. 'How they suffer. It is brutal. I have never seen anything like it,' wrote Sister Cathy Mellor.[2]

Sister Margaret Melrose has never forgotten those hectic days.

It was a frantic time for us, but we never gave much thought to what we were doing then, nor how tired we must have been. We just saw the long line of stretchers outside the operating theatre and carried on with moving them in for the surgeon and then taking down to the wards those pathetic looking men emerging from the operating theatre. What I remember most about those days is the way those wounded men who were conscious managed to raise a smile or make some sort of joke about it all. They were all so young. And many of them all so badly mutilated. All so brave. And so many died.[3]

The battle for Gallipoli, despite the valour of the British, Australian and New Zealand troops, soon became a struggle that everyone saw could never be won. It became more and more like the Western Front, with ill-planned attacks against heavily defended positions, as if few lessons had been learnt from previous failures. Casualty lists grew even longer.

In the torrid summer that made Gallipoli almost unbearable, malaria and dysentery took such a heavy toll that dead were piled in heaps that gave off a sickening stench. An epidemic looked so likely that medical staff urged General Birdwood to ask the Turks for a brief armistice. Hostilities were suspended for nine hours on 24 May as doctors, padres, orderlies and burial parties dug holes to get rid of the threat of a deadly epidemic.

Despite the efforts of medical and sanitary personnel, casualties from endemic sickness increased alarmingly. Clouds of fat black flies, soiled with all kinds of filth, swarmed throughout the trenches. They had feasted on dead and decomposing bodies, the open latrines and settled on food prepared by soldiers with little idea of food hygiene. Almost everybody had dysentery to some degree.

Nurses were horrified to see the state of those men evacuated from the beaches to their hospital ships. Surgeon Duncan Lorrimer of HMS *Baccante* recalled a time he went on board a transport ship bringing casualties to Mudros and saw casualties packed all over the ship in complete disorder. Wounds had not been dressed for two days and over them crawled plump yellow maggots replete from feasting on infected flesh. 'It made one ashamed of the Army that did not have enough nurses and doctors,' he said.

Sister Mary Fitzgibbon, QAIMNS, could never forget the men suffering from dysentery: 'Miserable, dehydrated and in terrible pain. It was pitiful to see them so weak and blood and water pouring out of them. We had medicine but we could do little for them.'

When the fierce heat of summer turned into a stormy autumn and quickly into a freezing winter, men without protective clothing in the trenches suffered further torments. In one snowstorm alone, 16,000 men reported sick with frostbite. Exposure killed 300.

Inevitably by the end of 1915 the new commander-in-chief came to the conclusion that his only course was to cut his losses and abandon the campaign altogether. It was no easy matter. With maximum secrecy, without lights and with smoking banned, men were withdrawn from the Suvla Bay line night after night until there were only thirty men left. These would run silently, with blankets wrapped round their boots, from one part of the line to another, firing rifles to make it appear that the defence was strong enough to deter a Turkish attack. The last troops to leave their positions, only 100 yards from the Turkish trenches, withdrew silently into the night to the quayside.

There, with nothing between them and the whole of the Turkish army, the last of the 138,000 defenders were taken off without the loss of one of them. Turks were still shelling Allied trenches as their previous occupants were moving silently along the embarkation piers. Nurses in their hospital ships had taken off the last of the wounded and were safely at sea.

Ironically the withdrawal, completed on 9 January 1916, was the most efficiently organized operation of the whole campaign. Behind them they left only their dead and a reputation among the Turks for bravery and fighting ability second to none.

Then the cost of that disastrous eight months' campaign was reckoned. British and Anzac casualties amounted to 214,000 and the French 47,000.

Though the Gallipoli campaign failed in its objectives the War Council had other plans for attacking Germany from the east. Already a second distracting sideshow against the Germans had been opened with its base at Salonika in northern Greece.

Once again British nurses were in action. Nurses of Number 1 General Hospital were sent from Port Said to Salonika for service with Australian and New Zealand troops. For some unknown reason they sailed in a troop and ammunition transport ship, the *Marquette*, instead of a hospital ship, the *Grantully Castle*, which was also sailing empty for Salonika.

On 19 October 1915 the *Marquette* was torpedoed within sight of Salonika and sank within seven minutes. When the ship tilted, lifeboats crashed into one another as they were being lowered, crushing some passengers, while others were thrown into the water. Of the twenty-six nursing sisters on board, ten were killed or drowned. The survivors returned to Egypt suffering from shock and exposure.

Nurses arriving at Salonika from the United Kingdom for this new campaign were very surprised to find they were bound for Serbia. 'Never for a moment did I ever imagine I should be writing home from the wilds of Serbia, when I joined the Army Nursing Service just before the war,' wrote Doris Dickson. 'I thought we nurses would be somewhere in France. I never really understood why we had been sent to Serbia.'[4]

Doris Dickson was not alone. To the British public Serbia was a small country somewhere south of Belgrade and responsible for the start of the war. No one seemed to know what was really happening there except for some terrible stories. The reasoning behind the campaign begins elsewhere.

German and Bulgarian troops had overrun most of Serbia in August 1914. After a period of reinforcement and regrouping, the Serbian army retaliated and pushed back the Austrian army on to its own soil, with losses of 40,000 men on the Austrian side.

Smarting over his army's defeat, the Austrian chief of staff, General Conrad von Hortzendorf, launched another attack on the Serbs in November 1914. In brutal fighting the two armies inflicted terrible casualties on each other before the Austrians were again pushed back behind their own borders. Now the German high command was worried about Austria's weakened plight and dispatched four German corps from France to bail out their inept allies.

In August 1915, Bulgaria declared war on Britain and France and joined forces with the Austrians against Serbia. The situation for the Serbs was now critical and they appealed to Britain for military help. Britain with her commitments on the Western Front could hardly afford to send men in large numbers but they had promised aid for Serbia and could not abandon an ally to her fate. Consequently in October 1915, an Anglo-French army landed at Salonika to take over the defence of Serbia.

Soon the British forces stationed in the south-east corner of Serbia successfully defended their lines against intermittent attacks from the German–Bulgarian force. Once the Allies had committed their troops to opposing the German–Bulgarian divisions, it was impossible to withdraw them.

The campaign became a much bigger affair than was generally realized in Britain. In the probing and patrolling of each other's lines, both sides inevitably suffered casualties. A steady stream of men suffering from gun-shot wounds and disease kept the nurses busy night and day. What made matters worse was that many of the doctors in the Serbian army had either died in the typhus epidemic earlier in the year or been killed in the battle of Kosovo. Some idea of the strength of British forces engaged and the casualties incurred can be seen from the fact that seventeen general hospitals, four stationary hospitals, five casualty clearing stations and two convalescent camps had to be established to deal with the sick and wounded.

Serving with these medical units were over 1,000 trained nurses. One of these was Albina Jane Pinninger, on the staff of the First British field hospital, a tented encampment situated near the Serbian town of Skopjie on the river Vardar.

Early in 1914 Albina Pinninger had been nursing as a civilian in a hospital on the outskirts of Belgrade. When the Bulgarians attacked Serbia she was attached to the 3rd Serbian army. She, together with what seemed like the whole of the population, retreated southwards through cruel and forbidding mountains, one high peak after another. Albina Pinninger could keep going only by telling herself that the next ridge would be the last, and not daring to think of the mountains ahead still to be climbed.[5]

As she trudged through the snow with a scarf wrapped round her head, leaving only a narrow gap for her eyes to peep through at the track ahead, it seemed to Albina as though the retreat would never end. However, the boom of the guns behind them was enough to remind the refugees to keep moving forward.

At last Albina Pinninger, along with eight British doctors and fifteen other nurses, reached Monastir (now Bitola). Incredibly, they had survived a hazardous journey of sixty miles on foot in atrocious blizzards. On the way fifteen out of their twenty pack mules died of hunger.

Further south in Salonika another drama was unfolding.

Nurses posted to a hospital there arrived in time to witness an event which tested the British Army's medical services to its utmost limit.

Early one morning in the summer of 1917, fire broke out in the Turkish quarter of Salonika and fanned by a strong breeze, spread rapidly through the old congested part of the city. Roaring flames engulfed the quaint ancient minarets and mosques. The back-street dwellings around the city centre went up in flames before the fire fighters and Allied troops managed to dowse them. By that time though, hundreds had been badly burnt and over 100,000 people made homeless.

The disaster triggered a great rallying of military and civilian services. Allied troops transported women and children to the safety of the countryside, while other army units patrolled the devastated areas preventing looting. Much to the surprise of the civilian population those poorly paid British infantrymen resisted the temptation to pick up valuable items left in empty property. Indeed they looked after them in a way that brought praise from the locals who returned.

Nurses came from nearby hospitals to take charge of medical centres in refugee camps. There, they treated more than just fire casualties. Once word got round to the more elderly of the refugees that kind nurses and doctors were in the vicinity, they flocked to the medical tents to have their chronic ailments treated. The willing and tender-hearted British nurses, then without many battle casualties to treat, hadn't the heart to turn them away.

A few months later, however, battle casualties began to fill the wards. Under a new French commander the Allied force attacked the Bulgars with all their available firepower.

British nurses moved forward with casualty clearing stations close to the front line, as the infantry maintained the momentum of their attack on all fronts. The Bulgarian forces at first defended every yard of their territory with fanatical desperation. They fought rearguard actions up the Struma Valley through Radomir and into Sofia itself. Casualties were heavy.

For this campaign in Macedonia and Serbia – called 'a wild goose chase' by British prime minister Herbert Asquith – 400,000 troops were committed. Out of them records show that the number of cases falling ill throughout the campaign was 481,000! Dysentery and malaria killed many of them or attacked them repeatedly.

Nurses too fell victim to the scourge of disease. Thirteen nurses died, two of them being killed in an air raid. On one of those raids nurses displayed some of the finest examples of courage and devotion to duty. Typical was their bravery on 27 February 1918, when German bombers made a low-level attack on Number 37 General Hospital, then attached to the Serbian army.

As bombs were dropping, Sisters Margaret Smith Dewar, Annie Rebecca Calhoun and Ethel Garrett of the QAIMNS Reserve rushed round the tented wards attempting to improvise some sort of cover for the patients. Sister Dewar was just placing a pillow to protect the head of a patient when a bomb exploded close to her in the ward and a piece of bomb casing pierced her chest as she knelt over the wounded soldier.

'The whole of the nursing staff behaved magnificently,' wrote the commanding officer in his unit war diary. 'Had Sister Dewar not risen to perform her act of protection it is probable that she herself would have escaped. The act showed complete disregard for her own safety. Her chief thought seems to have been for the safety of her patient.'

Sister Calhoun, in the same tent, was helping a patient who was unable to move himself, when she too was struck by a bomb splinter. She was fit enough, however, to go to the aid of Sister Dewar, who died in her arms. She then returned to support her helpless patient.

Sister Garrett rushed to the side of a patient with a compound fracture of the skull, caused by a bomb falling close to his tent. Having treated him she went to help a Serbian patient. Bombs continued to fall.

The gallantry of those nurses was recognized by the Crown Prince of Serbia, who awarded the Serbian Military Medal for Valour to Sisters Calhoun and Garrett. It was the first time such an honour had been bestowed on women. Many were the nurses, though, who gave their utmost when the need arose, not only when in the firing line but also through sheer overwork. Typical of this kind of self-sacrifice was the way in which Staff Nurse Jessie Ritchie of the QAIMNS with Number 26 Hospital in Salonika died of dysentery in 1916.

Her Matron wrote, in a letter to the British Journal of Nursing of 2 September 1916, that her death could be attributed to her devotion to duty. Most of her time was spent nursing enteric or dysentery. Characteristically her selfless nature meant that the care of her patients always took precedence over her need to rest when she herself was ill. In concluding her letter, Matron wrote: 'The Army Nursing Service is sadly poorer by her death. But what an incentive her beautiful memory is to all that is best in British womanhood.'[6]

Though but a few personal examples of the devotion to duty displayed by nurses in this theatre have been named here they stand for the whole of the army nursing service in Salonika. It is a sorry story, and little can be seen of all their efforts in that ancient Greek city today save for the rows of white crosses where 10,000 British soldiers lie buried in the military cemetery. Here and there one comes across the graves of those wartime army nursing sisters marked in the same way as the men around them. As one visitor to the Lambeth Road military cemetery in Salonika was heard to remark on seeing such a cross: 'What better escort could an army nurse want across the river?'

While no less than 1,066 trained nurses from British, Canadian and Australian armies, plus 224 VADs, were engaged in the Serbian campaign, other nurses were on active service in Italy.

At the outbreak of war in 1914, Italy had been hesitant to commit herself definitely to one or the other combatant powers. She had ties with Germany and Austria–Hungary, under a treaty agreed in 1882, but she was also reluctant to go to war against Britain, which had helped her in the past. She was also tempted to throw in her lot with Britain in the hope of being rewarded with possession of the Trentino and Trieste.

For the first eight months of the war Italy remained neutral, bargaining skilfully with both sides. In May 1915, however, she came to a decision and entered the war on the side of Britain and France. For the next year and a half she gave the Allies invaluable assistance by pinning down Austrian divisions on her frontiers with a series of courageous offensive actions by her prestigious mountain warfare troops.

British nurses soon became involved in this theatre of operations. It was a long and arduous campaign in the rugged, often snow-bound, Alps, through the valley of Isonzo and on the stony plateau of the Carso. Ill-equipped Italian troops fought with great courage, losing in these encounters over 280,000 men. Worse was to come. In the summer of 1917, the collapse of Russia left Germany and Austria free to mount a strong offensive against Italy.

Through the early morning mist of 24 October 1917, six German and nine Austrian divisions attacked at Caporetto in the mountains beyond Udine, towards the border with Austria. After a barrage of mustard-gas shells against which Italian respirators provided no protection, panic-stricken Italian infantry staggered out of their defensive positions in blind, choking confusion. Then came an artillery barrage of high-explosive shells, closely followed by fresh assault troops who advanced with machine-guns, hand grenades, flame throwers and small bombs filled with gas, which for the first time proved terribly effective. Despite heroic resistance of the Alpini troops, the Caporetto front crumbled.

Within twenty-four hours the Second Italian Army was, for practical purposes, destroyed. It reeled back almost to Venice before regrouping on the river Piave. In their defensive withdrawal the Italian army lost 10,000 dead and 30,000 wounded, while 295,000 men were prisoner. Now little was left to hold back the next Austrian advance.

The situation for the Allies was now grave. Italy had to actively engage Austrian and German troops to keep them away from the Western Front. In response to desperate appeals for help, the Allies rushed six French and five British divisions with their hospital facilities and nurses to reinforce the Italian army. They were just in time to hold the line on the Piave. In that bitter struggle British nurses serving under conditions of considerable danger and discomfort, often in mansions hastily converted for hospital use, made a great contribution.

Some of them had already opened a hospital when they arrived in December 1915 by taking over big hotels in Genoa, and as more nurses arrived in 1916 and early 1917, they went to staff casualty clearing stations and field hospitals nearer the front line in northern Italy and base hospitals at Arquata, Cremona and Bordighera.

Sister D. Hay, serving with a field ambulance unit in the Villa Trento, close to Gorizia in the mountainous region of the border with Slovenia, remembered the Caporetto disaster very well. In the weeks before the final battle she had seen the infantry going up to the firing line each day and at dusk saw them coming back in the ambulance cars.

For months on end from the windows of the mansion we used as a hospital, we could see Cormons and Gorizia being shelled constantly. At night the mountains were lit up by Austrian search-lights. Frequently we had to send two nurses at a time to the dressing station at Dolegna. They decided who was fit enough to make the journey back to us. We received thousands of wounded men to whom we gave coffee and bread and changed their dressings where necessary.

Many of them who had been up in the snow-covered mountain had frozen feet with toes and fingers dropping off and where their uniforms had frozen to sores on their bodies they were suppurating with pus, sometimes gangrenous. We always had a priest ready for them.

One evening, it was the 27th October 1917, an Italian officer rushed in and told us to leave at once. Hurriedly we got all the patients in ambulances or trucks and then had a frightening drive down the winding mountain roads. We came upon other camps also in hasty retreat with Italian troops setting fire to their ammunition dumps. We drove for hours and the roads became choked with people fleeing with as much of their worldly goods as they could load onto mule carts and hand-pulled trolleys. It was heart-rending to see the dead and dying lying by the roadside. And there was so little we could do for the soldiers whose lungs were so badly damaged with gas. There were horses too that had to be shot because of gas. Horses had gas masks like nose bags for feed which gave some protection but none at all for the eyes. Officers were told to draw imaginary lines between the eyes and opposite ears of the injured horse and where they crossed was the place for the revolver muzzle. The horse dropped immediately the trigger was pulled. They looked so pitiful as their forelegs folded.

All day and the next we drove desperately trying to get to the bridge at Tagliamento before it was blown up to delay the enemy's advance. The road then became too choked with people walking to continue driving so we had to abandon the car and walk also. The rain was torrential and we were soaked to the skin but at last we came to the river. As we got closer to it we saw people were begin-ning to panic and rush to get across the bridge spanning the swollen torrent. There were terrible sights of men and women fighting and some falling into the swirling, muddy river. It was a bizarre scene as people, packed alongside gun carriages, ox-carts and other transport, jostled their way across. There was even one old lady sitting upright in a landau driven by a coachman.

The confusion and congestion on the road was horrific. Rumours went round that the war was over and the only thing troops and

civilians wanted was to get home or to relatives away from the
advancing German and Austrian divisions. Panic cries that enemy
cavalry had been sighted caused villagers en route to turn out of
their houses and join the rush for the bridges and roads to the south.
Fugitives looted as they ran.

As daylight came we were tired out and thirsty. We stopped at a
farmhouse where we asked for water and were given both water and
wine. The farmer was so kind and his wife would take no money. We
had just left the farm when an Austrian plane bombed the house and
wrecked one side completely.[7]

At last the nurses came to the railway station at Casarso. There
were five trains waiting there. They boarded one that set off but
stopped after a mile. Starving soldiers were on the line and jumped
on the train to loot bread, sacks of flour and half carcasses of meat
which they carried into the fields and began to roast over open fires.
Other soldiers on the train, who told the nurses they had not eaten
anything for four days, cut pieces of meat and ate it raw. Sister Hay
and her colleagues tucked into tins of salmon and dry bread. By sunset
that day they reached Pordanone, but even there they were not
considered safe from the great retreat and went on to Padua.

It was only at Padua that Sister Hay saw what was in the basket
that her friend, Sister Gibson, had been carrying so carefully. It was
her cat.

The nurses went by train via Paris to London. There on 7
November 1917 they were met by the press and photographers, who
were more interested in taking pictures of the cat in the basket than
the returning nurses.

On the front line in Italy, the Italian 3rd Army held the German-
Austrian forces on the River Tagliamento. Britain and France
promised substantial aid in arms and men.

Part of that 'substantial aid' consisted of further drafts of nursing
sisters. During this period nurses were working hard in cold hospitals
– Italy had no coal mines and was short of fuel – but never again were
they overrun by the enemy. Having for three years suffered the presence of enemy troops on her soil, Italy was ready in the autumn of
1918 to take the offensive. On the anniversary of Caporetto, with
twenty-one divisions of infantry and 1,600 guns, they attacked the
Austrian army with such overwhelming ferocity that it crumbled and
surrendered.

Italy's contribution to final victory in the First World War has never
been fully recognized. The war had cost the country nearly 2 million

casualties – 460,000 dead, 947,000 wounded and the remainder prisoners. All told, Italy lost more men as a proportion of its population than any other continental power involved in the conflict.

For the nurses in Italy, conditions improved with the summer of 1918. Until the final offensive and even then British nurses had little to contend with apart from the occasional air raid. Consequently, nurses working behind the lines were able to enjoy life in the sunny Mediterranean climate. This was especially true for those stationed in Taranto, in the south of Italy, where the Red Cross social club provided opportunities for sport and social activities in the sun.

For all those nurses it was a well-deserved break.

# 9 Prickly Heat and Pestilence

'If your head is wax, don't walk in the sun.'
Benjamin Franklin, 1706–1790

It was to even sunnier climes in February 1916 that nurses were being dispatched in ever increasing numbers to look after thousands of sick and wounded men brought to Egypt from minor campaigns in the Middle East.

These nurses not only served in base hospitals in Egypt, but proved themselves to be adaptable to a wide variety of conditions on hospital ships, ambulance trains and motor ambulances by means of which the wounded were conveyed from campaigns in Palestine, Gallipoli, Salonika, Mesopotamia and East Africa.

Within ten days of the landing at Gallipoli nurses in Egypt were looking after more than 16,000 wounded and sick, under very difficult conditions. True, some preparation had been made for heavy casualties – two general hospitals had been sent to Egypt – but nursing sisters had not yet come from Britain. As a stopgap, local nurses were employed from hospitals in Cairo but soon QA nursing sisters with more fighting troops began to arrive from Britain.

At that time, the control of Egypt was strategically crucial for the survival of the British Empire. It safeguarded the Suez Canal and therefore the short route to India and the Persian Gulf. A quarter of a million men were kept in Egypt to guard the Suez Canal from the threat of another Turkish attack, such as the one launched in 1915.

Nurses too were on the way to Mesopotamia (soon to become Iraq in 1921). When Turkey joined Germany and the Central Powers in the war against Britain on 1 November 1914, the British army had only one brigade in the Persian Gulf, located on Abadan Island. Its role was to protect the pipelines of the Anglo-Persian Oil Company.

A few nurses, drawn mainly from the Indian Army nursing service, were stationed there.

Britain hoped that the Arabs, known to be smouldering under Turkish rule, would rebel and so augment the British forces going to Mesopotamia, but this failed to happen.

Abadan was not a suitable base for a large garrison, which was clearly going to be necessary given the weight of wartime commitments. So on 22 November 1914, the British brigade moved north and seized Basra, the main port at the head of the Persian Gulf.

British nursing sisters moved to Basra to staff numbers 23 and 32 general hospitals early in 1916, as soon as two divisions arrived from India's north-west frontier to strengthen the garrison. There they were kept busy caring for war wounded and hundreds suffering from malaria and dysentery.

Sister Bond of the QAIMNS recalled the problems that these diseases presented to nurses at Basra. In a letter to the *Nursing Record* of July 1916 she wrote: 'Only those who have lived in a mosquito infested country, know the torment as well as the dangers of the bites (not stings) of those pestilential insects – intractable ulcers, exquisitely painful boils, not to mention malaria, which follow in their wake.'

Swarms of mosquitoes added to the discomfort of troops on the Tigris. The hungry insects bit through clothes to get at moist skin.

The treatment of dysentery was difficult and worrisome. Nurses realized that best results were obtained when treatment began as soon as possible, but usually soldiers would put up with the diarrhoea and other symptoms for three or four days before reporting sick. Then their strength and resistance were low and their blood saturated with toxins. If possible treatment would be with ipecacuanha, emulsion of castor oil, sulphate of magnesia or a similar saline, such as Glauber's Salts.

Unfortunately medication was not always available and also it was very difficult to get sick men back to hospital. The situation angered the assistant director of medical services so much that he wrote to newspapers back home:

Accommodation to get sick men to hospital is shockingly bad, in fact hopeless. Field Ambulances are looking after 500 patients instead of 50, for anything from a week to three weeks instead of for a few days. The Field Ambulance itself has lost a third of its staff due to sickness because they won't send transport to us with trained personnel. Patients suffer agony here instead of being in a proper hospital. It makes me boil with righteous indignation.[1]

With hindsight it is easy to say that the British advance should have stopped at Basra and the high command should have resisted the lure of advancing to capture Baghdad, but unfortunately for the British Tommy and the nurses who looked after him, the plans changed to the ambitious one of driving northwards to seize the country's capital and centre of its transportation network.

The newly appointed commander-in-chief of British troops was General Townshend, a highly ambitious man said to have one eye permanently on the promotion ladder. He was attracted to the idea of capturing the glittering prize of Baghdad. He decided to begin his advance northwards towards that city. At first all went well. Turkish troops seemed to fall back in disarray as British divisions struggled to make progress through the peculiar swampy, fever-ridden terrain of the Tigris–Euphrates valley. He soon discovered that few places in the world are as hot as the central plains of Mesopotamia: daytime temperatures regularly reached 120°F.

Nevertheless, his troops managed to advance ninety miles to capture Amara on 3 June. Closely behind the infantry divisions came seven nursing sisters with their matron. For them, travelling by paddle steamer up the river Tigris, it was a memorable journey.

At Qurnah, where the Tigris and Euphrates meet, date palms, willows and poplars lined the banks of the river. Flocks of birds, particularly grouse and partridge, flew from the green marshland. Sister Iris Wilkinson wrote in a letter home: 'We passed where the Garden of Eden was and even saw the Tree of Knowledge itself.'

At Amara they joined the Rawalpindi Hospital, mobilized on the north-west frontier of India. In charge of them was a superintendent of the Indian nursing service.

With his success in capturing Amara, Townshend was deceived. He assumed the Turks had no wish to fight, but in fact the Turkish commander had decided there was little strategic value in defending Amara and withdrew to regroup in greater strength further north. Now when Townshend pushed his weary troops northwards they met fierce resistance and casualties streamed into the hospital at Amara from battles fought around Kut and Ktesiphon. By the time the wounded reached nurses in base hospital wards they were in a pitiable condition having travelled more than 200 miles in open barges with poor sanitation and little cover from the heat of the sun.

In addition to fighting the enemy, the British forces had to contend with excessive exposure to heat and with smallpox, cholera, malaria, blackwater fever, dysentery and all the other diseases and discomforts brought by flies. A veritable plague of flies. Soon so many men were falling sick that Number 23 tented stationary hospital was extended to provide 1,000 beds.

One nurse gave a vivid picture of what it was like when she described a visit to the officers' mess of the 2/7th battalion of the Gurkha Regiment. Before the meal began, the small party of nurses there was treated to a unique method of getting rid of flies. A mess orderly tied a piece of string from the ridge pole of the tent upon which flies settled in their thousands. Then, filling his mouth with paraffin he struck a match and blew a flame quickly at his target. There was a tremendous buzzing, followed by a quick dusting-off of the corpses lying on the boxes that served as dinner tables. On these the orderly then solemnly laid tin plates and cutlery.

It was a terrible country in which to wage war. Mile upon mile of desert scrub stretched as far as the eye could see. The intense, shimmering heat produced mirages, which made the task of observation posts difficult. Trees for shade were scarce, and the only vegetation was an occasional date palm or patch of thorny scrub. When the snows melted in the highlands, rivers and streams broke their banks and vast areas of the lowland regions were completely flooded. Where not under water the land was turned into a thick, glutinous mud, worse even than that of Flanders. War correspondents' photographs showed troops wading knee-deep through the muddy water.

Transportation of rations and ammunition was extremely difficult for roads rarely existed and where found were in an appalling state of disrepair. Carriage of goods was mainly confined to rivers. Small wonder the physical and mental health of the fighting battalions in forward areas was so below par.

Many nurses found themselves treating for the first time men with vascular collapse due to heatstroke. The onset of the condition, in previously apparently healthy soldiers, was surprisingly sudden and dramatic.

Soldiers were admitted in a state of delirium and coma that apparently had come on after a short period of headaches, during which they often wandered about dizzy as if drunk. Some vomited, others had difficulty in speaking and swallowing. All of them suffered from an intense thirst.

Closely allied to heatstroke was heat exhaustion, in which soldiers started with a headache, a feeling of nausea and mild vomiting. Some reported sick with spots before their eyes and a ringing in their ears. They complained of feeling very thirsty and of vomiting after taking a drink of water. Indeed, the problem for soldiers in Mesopotamia was that their intake of water rarely kept pace with their perspiration, leaving them with a deficit medical textbooks termed 'voluntary dehydration' – but it was far from voluntary given the daily water-bottle ration on which each soldier had to manage.

It was alarming for those nurses caring for such patients for the first time. Men had very high pulse rates, as rapid as 130 beats a minute and a shallow breathing rate of thirty times a minute. The discomfort of heatstroke patients and the problems for nurses and orderlies were made worse by incontinence.

In extreme cases patients developed a form of epilepsy, with violent muscular twitching of arms and legs. Many died simply through heat exhaustion; among them were seven senior officers, one of whom was Sir Victor Horsley. He had already reported to the War Office the appalling failures in medical arrangements due to defective transport and also due to the unsatisfactory relations between the British government's financial departments and the Indian government's medical services. 'There's nothing but the foulest store barges and steamers to be used for taking the sick and wounded back to base hospitals,' he wrote.[2]

Summing up his report of medical mismanagement, Sir Victor put his finger directly on the cause, one which was to recur time after time in the history of British wartime medical services: 'Financial terrorism in times of peace,' by the party in power. This referred to the way politicians saved money in peace time by cutting expenditure on the armed forces. It was ironic that Sir Victor would himself fall victim to that terrorism and to the heatstroke that killed him.

Ice and fans, with which overheated patients could have been cooled, were in short supply. The best that some wards could do was to spray patients with the coolest water they could find, wrap them in wet sheets and have them fanned vigorously to produce cooling by evaporation. Some hospitals employed a *punkah-wallah* to waft and move the air with make-shift fans. Fortunate wards had a motor-driven fan. Not surprisingly for veteran soldiers who had served their time in India, the Arab boys employed as *punkah-wallahs* were also such expert thieves that they could slip the prized red army blanket off the bed of a sleeping patient without even waking him.

Nurses had to be extra vigilant with all their personal underwear and kit.

Working in the wards was particularly difficult. Nurses, oddly dressed in their gum-boots and topees, plodded through mud from bed to bed working from early morning until very late at night. Despite being dead-beat, few of them could manage a good night's sleep. They were plagued with flies, fleas, bugs, and vicious mosquitoes. Within a few months some sisters were in such a run-down condition that they were evacuated for rehabilitation to hospitals in India.

In Mesopotamia, life was so difficult that nursing sisters and soldiers of all ranks often wondered why they were there. Why indeed! Many believed the British Cabinet wanted to capture Baghdad to divert public attention from the Gallipoli misadventure. But what had Baghdad to offer? A city of minarets, mosques, magic carpets and thieves; a mixture of splendour and abject poverty. How would its capture help the Allied war effort?

General Townshend was not dismayed, however. Here was his opportunity to show what he could do, to make a name for himself. He certainly made a name, but not one to be remembered with pride. Many years earlier his name had been displayed in banner headlines in the national press after he survived a 46-day siege on the north-west frontier of India. But that was now long ago. He would have to do something more remarkable. So he decided to push on towards Baghdad. Permission was given for the enterprise in a peculiarly half-hearted telegram: 'the Commander-in-Chief may march on Baghdad if he is satisfied the force he has available is sufficient for the operation'.

Advancing in terrible conditions, with the hot wind whipping up the sand into a thick fog, British divisions got within sixteen miles of Baghdad when they came under intense fire from Turks defending the fortified ruins of ancient Ctesiphon, once the southernmost tip of the Roman Empire.

British and Indian divisions were beaten back. General Townshend lost 4,500 men of whom 800 were killed. Casualties poured into hospital wards after an awful journey from the front line. There was no chance now of Townshend reaching Baghdad, for another 30,000 troops had now been rushed to reinforce the fresh Turkish divisions who had been lying in wait for the arrival of the exhausted British troops.

Thus the British Tommy began a long retreat down the Tigris valley. At Kut-al-Imara, Townshend stopped and prepared to dig in and wait for a relief column. So began one of the longest sieges in British military history. Soon rations became almost exhausted. Soldiers resorted to eating their horses and even toasted starlings. Starvation took its toll. On 1 April, Colonel Maule noted in his diary, 'The men are dying off fast now from starvation, scurvy, pneumonia.' Of his colleague Wood, he added a short note in the stiff-upper-lip mode: 'after recovering splendidly when his arm was blown off, he has died of jaundice. A good fellow!'

On 22 April, Lieutenant Bell Syer noted in his diary: 'We are down to starvation rations now.' A relief force approached slowly. One of its members, Captain Dawson, wrote in his diary: 'Cholera has started. We had to march in the heat of the day to relieve trenches. We lie and gasp all day under a blanket which we put up to keep off the sun which it does indifferently.'

Altogether, 23,000 died in futile attempts to break through Turkish lines to relieve Townshend's troops. With his men nearing absolute starvation, Townshend surrendered. Some 13,000 British prisoners left Kut and were flogged by Turks on a forced march across the desert to prisoner-of-war camps. On the way 60 per cent of them died. General Townshend was put on a train to Constantinople, where he was housed in accommodation the Turks thought fit for a general – a palace with two servants – and given a yacht for his entertainment. They say he never more enquired about his troops.

During this time more and more nurses were arriving at Basra and then at Amara. By 1917 conditions there improved for them. The Red Cross brought in 'comforts' – cigarettes, parcels and letters from home. Occasionally, too, concert parties even came to give impromptu performances in the wards.

On 8 January 1917, Number 65 General Hospital arrived at Basra with sixty-one nurses, half of them fully trained sisters of the QAIMNS and the others of the VAD. Soon Number 33 General Hospital was set up with 500 beds, in an old liquorice factory at Makinaon. At Nasiriya, on the banks of the Euphrates north of Basra, a large British and Indian hospital opened for those sick and wounded fit enough to travel by train down to Basra.

Eventually, as if to redeem the series of humiliating defeats, 100,000 troops were committed to the campaign in Mesopotamia, and in March 1917, British and Indian divisions took Baghdad.

Six weeks later, nurses of hospitals that had operated in tents began to move into Baghdad. Five military hospitals were set up in the city: two stationary hospitals, an isolation, an officers' hospital and an officers' convalescent depot.

Nurses then enjoyed the novelty of shopping in the narrow streets crowded with bazaars. But those nurses posted to Number 23 Stationary British Hospital shuddered as they discovered it was a former Turkish military hospital – verminous, filthy, and needing cleansing, delousing, and fumigating before nurses, orderlies, or patients could stay there.

VAD nurse, Eleanor Pickering, was told by matron to take good care of a sergeant major with malaria. He looked at her and said to himself, 'I'm going to marry that girl'. Six months later he did. 'We had forty-eight glorious years together', said Eleanor

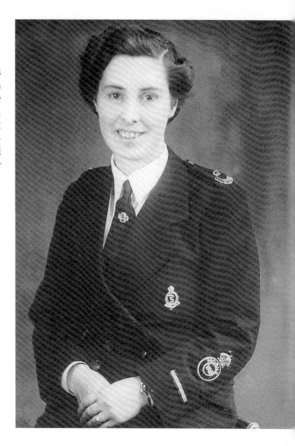

Eleanor Pickering (*front left*) at a reunion of VAD nurses from Catterick Military Hospital in April 2000. 'There used to be 200 of us meeting but now there's just sixteen. Like old soldiers we don't die, we just fade away', said Eleanor

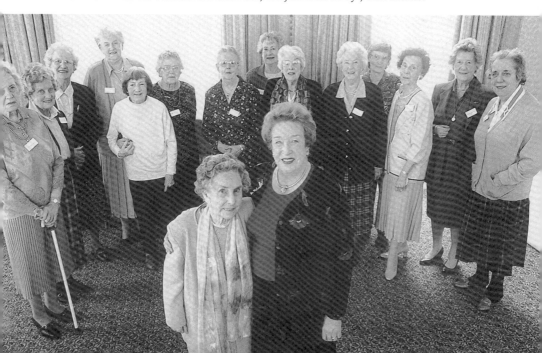

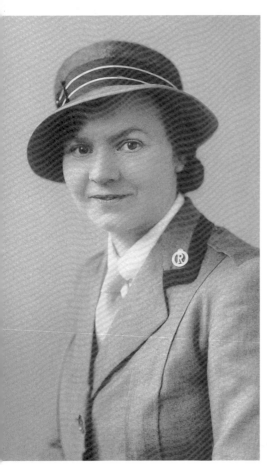

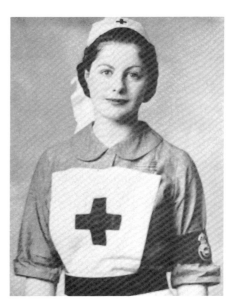

Helen Vlasto (later Long) in VAD uniform at Royal Naval Hospital, Haslar, early in World War Two

Sister Violet Bath (later Leather), and five other volunteer sisters, were called to matron's office and told to 'volunteer' for QAIMNS reserve. One of the six, Sister Lee, was killed on active service in Italy

Sister Marie Sedman QAIMNS (now Floyd-Norris) taken in Normandy, June 1944

Marie Floyd-Norris with the German Iron Cross given to her in a military hospital in Normandy

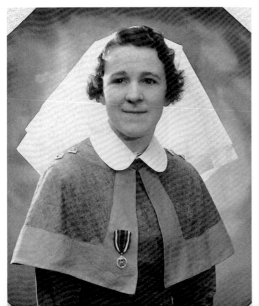

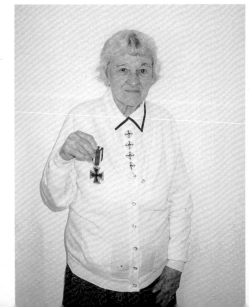

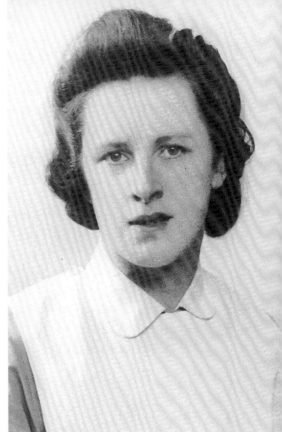

Nurse Joan Ottaway at the time
of the Coventry blitz

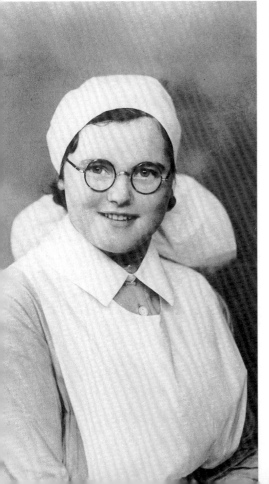

Gladys Spencer Crichton nursing
during the Coventry blitz

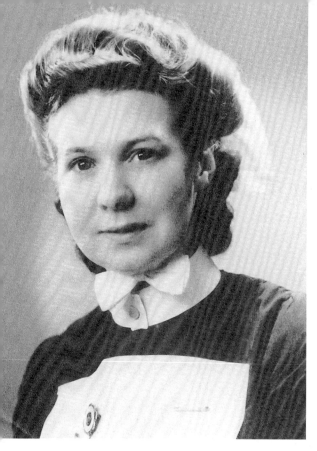

Edna Viner, 17-year-old
probationary nurse at the
Coventry and Warwickshire
Hospital during the heavy raids of
November 1940

VAD nurses trained by the Red Cross wore their emblem on hospital uniforms.
VAD nurses trained by St John Ambulance had a plain white uniform. Nursing
sister of the QAIMNS seen on right of ATS group

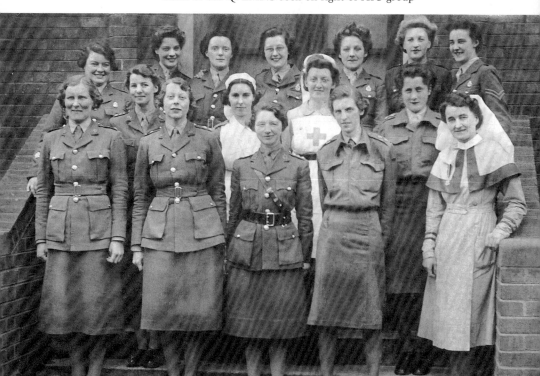

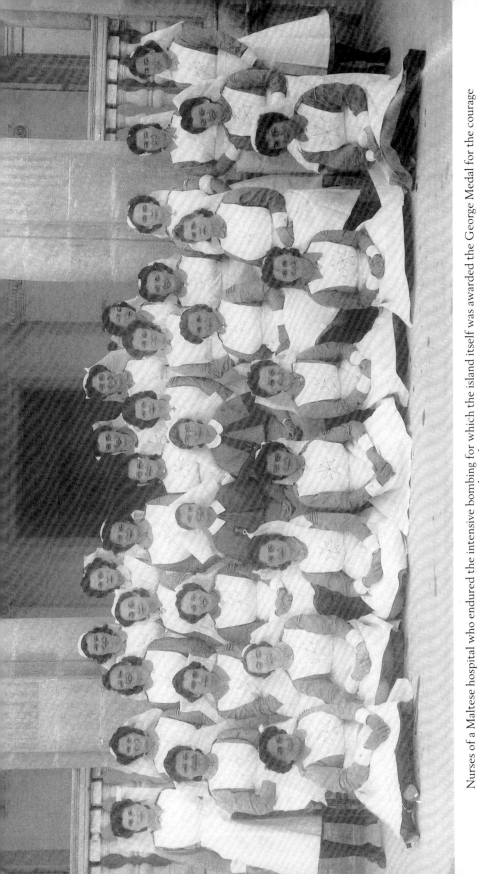

Nurses of a Maltese hospital who endured the intensive bombing for which the island itself was awarded the George Medal for the courage shown by everyone

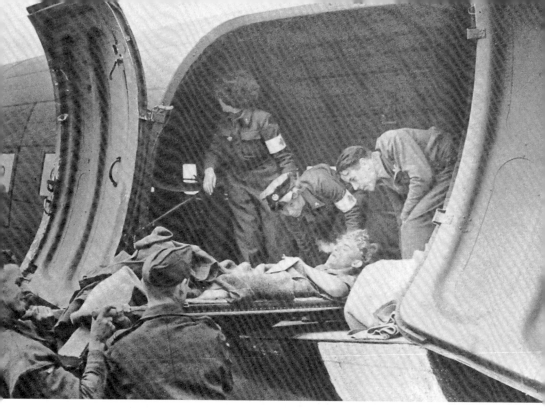

WAAF nursing orderly, Myra Roberts, receiving wounded on to an RAF air evacuation aircraft from a beach landing strip in Normandy shortly after D-Day

Supervision of patients on the flight back to the UK

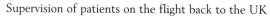

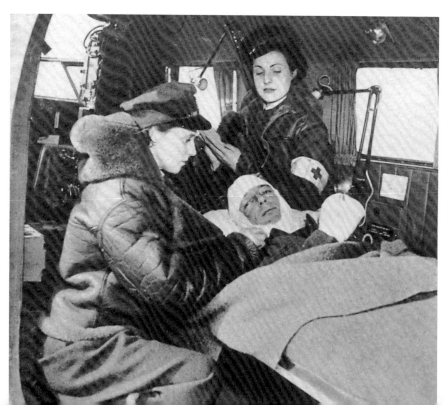

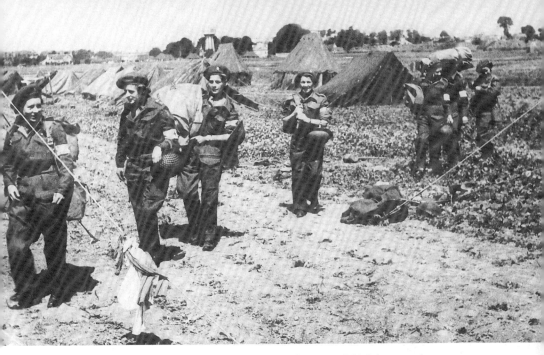

QAIMNS nursing sisters arriving in Normandy, June 1944 (photograph courtesy of the Imperial War Museum, London)

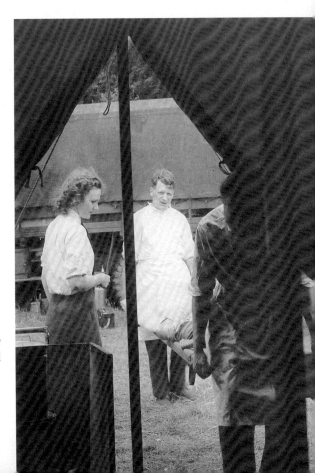

Casualties arriving at an RAF mobile field hospital

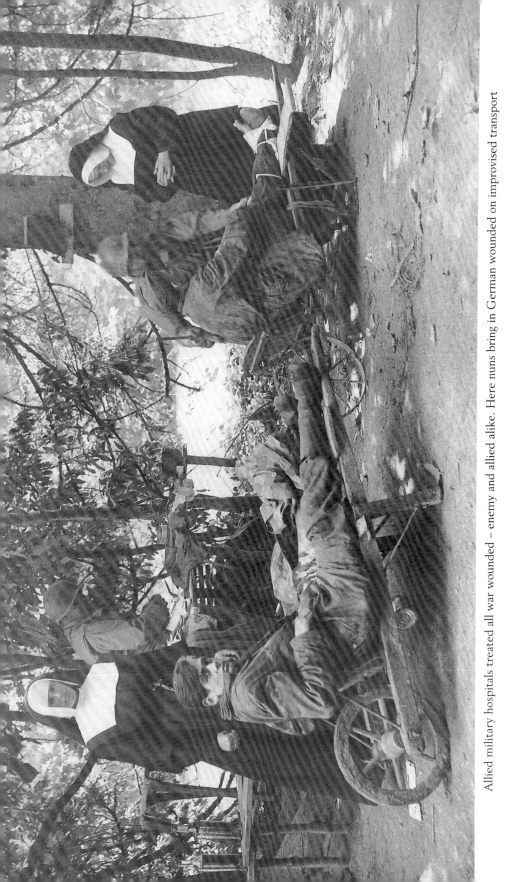

Allied military hospitals treated all war wounded – enemy and allied alike. Here nuns bring in German wounded on improvised transport

Living conditions for the nurses improved after they took over some of the cooler, flat-roofed houses. There were few patients and so nurses could take local leave in Baghdad.

Success in Mesopotamia, however, made little impact on the progress of the war on the Western Front, though newspapers in Britain tended to make much of the victory. A minor gain was at least something in such a disappointing year for the Allies.

At that time another branch of the British army was engaged in fighting Germany's ally Turkey in Palestine, and the nurses, as usual, were with them. Its first engagements were almost as catastrophic as those in the Dardanelles. After fierce fighting at Gaza, defended by a Turkish garrison of 400 warriors entrenched behind natural stockades of tightly clamped thorny cactus hedges, British forces had to withdraw. Most of the wounded went by hospital train to Egypt.

Apart from treating the usual battlefield wounds, nurses also came across apparently simple cactus pricks that had turned into serious cases of septicaemia causing abscesses in various parts of the body. Patients came into hospital with a high temperature, sweating profusely and shivering at the same time. In extreme cases, pain in joints and muscles became severe, and in those days when sulpha drugs and antibiotics were not available patients often died.

A month after the failure of British troops to take Gaza, General Murray launched a second attack. This was again repulsed, at a cost of 6,500 British casualties. Beset on all sides by failure, the British prime minister, Lloyd George, faced the situation in a time-honoured way by sacking the general officer commanding, in this case Murray, and appointing a new one, General Allenby, a man who had his own history of failure. He had incurred Haig's wrath with his lack of success at Arras in 1917. He came to Palestine with precise instructions from Lloyd George: 'Take Jerusalem!'

The capture of Jerusalem would boost British morale and shatter that of the Ottoman Empire. A victory over the Turks would make up for defeats on the Western Front. But the way to the Holy City was barred by an elaborate defence in depth, over twenty miles of linked weapon pits and trenches.

Allenby enlisted the help of pro-British Arab desert tribesmen organized by 29-year-old Colonel T.E. Lawrence. His men, experts in desert guerilla warfare, struck hard at Turkish columns, ambushing them and then disappearing into the desert.

Meanwhile Allenby assembled a British force of 80,000 men. They attacked the Turks at Beersheba to capture the fresh water wells and then defeated the Turks on the Judean Hills before Jerusalem. That victory was Britain's only success in 1917, but it came at the usual price. Casualties kept nurses fully employed.

To cope with them all, emergency hospitals were established in Egypt. Casualties came to them in small ships converted in to hospital carriers, but without the comforts of hospital ships. Wounded men suffered greatly before arriving in base hospitals. There the nurses, far from the improvised casualty clearing stations of the battle zones, could settle into an almost peacetime routine, as Lillian Lester described in letters home:

> We made the most of our time there when we were off duty, visiting the Great Pyramid of Giza. We felt like the rich tourists of old going into those famous hotels of Shepheard's and the Continental. I must say we felt a little bit nervous pushing our way through the crowded bazaar quarter of the *Mouski*, but we were young then and didn't worry much.
>
> Today I look at those old black and white photographs, taken on a box Brownie camera, showing a group of us sitting on camels, and I ask myself, did it all really happen?[3]

When the fighting around Jerusalem subsided, the Holy City was entered in a most remarkable way. General Sir Richard Allenby simply walked through the Jaffa Gate accompanied only by his personal staff and the commanders of the French and Italian detachments. The contrast between his entry and the bombastic peacetime entry of the Kaiser twenty years before was evident to all. He came as a deliverer not a conqueror.

British Forces with their medical officers and nurses then advanced from Jerusalem northwards with a mixed British and Indian force and by October entered Damascus (Dimashq). Now three Turkish armies simply disappeared. Turkey was out of the war, and the Ottomn Empire disintegrating.

Nurses serving in quieter hospital wards then, looking back on their days in the Balkans with all the discomforts of mosquitoes, mud and enemy shellfire, thought life in Egypt truly idyllic. Yet twenty-two nursing sisters and VADs died during that brief sojourn there. Some of them lost their lives serving in hospital ships sunk by enemy action even though those ships displayed Red Cross markings conspicuously.

Such was their vulnerability that a good number of these hospital ships were disguised with grey paint towards the end of the war, so as to make them indistinguishable from the merchant ships.[4]

The most serious loss of hospital shipping then was that of the magnificent 50,000-ton, White Star cruise liner *Britannic*. Built to replace the *Titanic*, which sank on her maiden voyage in April 1912, the *Britannic* was fitted out specifically as a hospital ship and dispatched for duty in the Mediterranean. Ironically, its fate was almost identical to that of the *Titanic*, for it was on its first voyage to collect a full complement of wounded from Gallipoli that it was holed by a U-boat's torpedo in the Aegean Sea, It went down as quickly as its illustrious predecessor had done.

Fortunately, no patients were on board and the nurses and medical personnel all survived to staff other hospital ships in the area. These were busy ferrying casualties from the Balkan and Middle East theatres of operations to Cairo, which despite one of the hottest and driest climates of the world was still able to provide comfortable hospital conditions in which wounds healed well.

From the ports, hospital trains conveyed sick and wounded to base hospitals. Accommodation on the trains was modified through experience at the request of nurses and medical officers to provide a through corridor, so that doctors and nurses could walk from one end of the train to the other without having to wait for a stop. Each train usually had three nursing sisters, for each of whom a sleeping cabin and a dining space was provided. Train duty was one which most nursing sisters got to like, for they had more independence than when serving in a stationary hospital and life was far more interesting.

There was no time for boredom. The routine kept everyone busy, not only during the journey but after patients had been delivered: all bed linen had to be changed, wards scrubbed and everything made ready for the next journey.

With the cessation of hostilities in Palestine, nursing sisters were available for posting to other theatres of operations. Many went to German East Africa, where the climate was even hotter and more pestilential than anything yet encountered by nurses. Every pool and swamp posed a hazard to health. Death lurked in the muddy waters.

On arrival most nurses went to the big hospital at Dar-es-Salaam, where nursing duties were shared between British army nurses and the VAD nurses, whose blue South African uniform got them known locally as the 'bluebirds'. Patients in the wards were mainly those suffering from malaria, rather than from bush warfare.

At one time twenty-one out of the sixty-three nurses staffing the hospital themselves succumbed to severe malarial fever. The symptoms were easily recognized. Victims bitten by anopheline mosquitoes reported sick with shivering; they had a flushed, dry skin and bright eyes. Most of them sweated profusely but not all. Many felt sick and were vomiting.

Attacks of malaria lasted longer for some than for others and the likelihood of a relapse was high. Some men in the 84th British Hospital at Dar-es-Salaam had been through fifteen to twenty bouts of malarial fever.

Associated with malaria and believed at that time to be brought on by quinine was the even more serious disease of blackwater fever. The mortality rate of this much feared condition varied from 20 to 30 per cent of all cases. Victims soon learnt to spot the dreaded signs in their urine. It gradually grew darker in colour over the course of a few hours, turning dark red and almost black. The treatment in hospital was one of absolute rest with intravenous transfusions of glucose, saline and plasma.

Nurses and soldiers who managed to avoid the more serious conditions had nevertheless to endure the discomfort of prickly heat and sunburn. Prickly heat with irritating skin eruptions was extremely common, even afflicting men and women who took great care with personal hygiene. Some doctors thought its cause was to do with the way that sweat-gland ducts became clogged by swollen skin layers, and it was particularly noticeable in men and women who tended to be overweight. Skin around folds of fat was severely affected. Men suffered more than women.

The trouble with such skin eruptions came with the itching and the consequent, almost involuntary scratching that broke the skin. Invariably, this caused a secondary infection.

Prickly heat tended to appear in those parts of the soldier's body in close contact with webbing belts around the waist or the straps of small packs rubbing over the shoulders. Apart from the risks of secondary infection, prickly heat also affected the general health of sufferers through loss of sleep and psychological reactions to the intolerable itching.

The best treatment, of course, was rest in cool surroundings. Then skin changes disappeared slowly and a full recovery could be made. In East Africa such a luxury was not possible.

What appeared to be of minor importance then but forty years later produced a good deal of anxiety were the effects of sunburn, called, in its extreme state, acute solar dermatitis. Soldiers took little care of their skin and often sunbathed to get an attractive tan to show off back home. The severity of sunburn depended upon whether the skin exposed was a delicate fair kind or a darker one. Skin once burnt tended to burn more easily on further exposure.

Lillian Lester recalled treatment for sunburn.

If a soldier came in with a badly burnt back we used to clean the area carefully with calamine lotion and then cover the affected part with calamine compresses. We had to be especially careful with blisters so as to avoid secondary infections. I think we nurses suffered less than the men because of the cosmetic creams and face powders we used which gave some protection. No one was conscious then how 'sunburn' could turn into cases of skin cancer some forty years later, as it did with some of those nurses. Soreness of sunburn was then more of an annoyance, under military law a 'self-inflicted wound', but rarely was anyone charged with that offence.

By the end of March 1918 in East Africa, with few battle casualties being admitted to the 84th General Hospital, nurses were kept busy dealing mainly with the sick and accident injuries. What becomes increasingly obvious in accounts of all these wartime nurses serving under such a wide variety of conditions is the magnificent way they adjusted to them all.

# 10 Carnage Incomparable

'It was like trying to bite through a steel door with badly fitting false teeth.'[1]

Marshal Joseph Joffre, French commander-in-chief

On 22 February 1916 dawn broke over Verdun with a mighty bombardment. It went on for the next eight hours. Quickly, nurses in the hospital at Le Petit Monthairon, four miles south of Verdun, were overwhelmed by a flood of casualties. French divisions defending the salient of Verdun were decimated. The main French hospitals, and smaller ones to take the overflow, were already established in local châteaux to receive casualties until field ambulance convoys could take them to the railhead at Revigny.

That night, VAD Winifred Kenyon left the operating theatre in a château close to the railhead, to see what the nurses and doctors were looking at so excitedly in the night sky. Shells were bursting round a silver cigar-shaped zeppelin caught in a searchlight's beam. Suddenly the zeppelin turned pink, then burst into bright flames and crumpled slowly to the ground leaving a trail of fire. Among the blazing frame-work on the ground, bodies could be seen.[2]

This was a critical time in the history of air warfare. Hitherto light aircraft had been used solely as observation posts, but now intercep-tor aircraft, fighters, were flying to shoot down reconnaissance aircraft. Those same aircraft were also used as bombers and piloted often by former infantry officers partially disabled in the war. Their life expectancy as a pilot was even shorter than that of an infantry subaltern – a very few weeks.

In the battles for Verdun casualties kept operating theatres in all hospitals, including that of Winifred Kenyon, working all hours. But despite the horrific number of wounded and dead, French high command would not countenance any withdrawal. 'Ils ne passeront pas,' promised General Pétain and the French infantry fought to keep the general's vow. The citadel town of Verdun was an emotionally hallowed symbol, standing for the mother country that French troops would defend whatever the cost. Which is just what German army commander von Falkenhayn had foreseen. When the French forces had been bled white he expected British divisions to fall into the same trap by attacking to take the pressure off Verdun. They too would then be pulverized. And pulverized they were.

At the beginning of the Verdun battle, British troops were holding a supposedly quiet part of the line. However, British commanders launched constant small offensives to ensure that German divisions opposite to their lines could not go to reinforce those attacking the French at Verdun.

What British commanders did not know was that German engineers opposite them were busy strengthening defences, making underground shelters forty feet deep and tunnels in which infantry and machine-guns could be sheltered safely during heavy Allied shelling. It was against these well-prepared positions that British battalions were frittered away in offensive actions that the commander of the French armies, General Joseph Joffre, called 'grignotage', a gnawing-away of German manpower with the ultimate aim of forcing the enemy out into the open.

To say this was a strange period in the war would be an understatement. Nurses heard tales from wounded soldiers of German and British troops using the same well for water; of soldiers swimming within sight of each other in the river Somme; and even of German and British officers carousing together over wine in opposing dugouts. Yet repeated offensives were still launched, filling the wards of base hospitals.

Nevertheless, so confident of ultimate victory was Haig through the tactics of attrition that he assured *The Times* war correspondent that once the Allies had stocked up a massive reserve of artillery shells they would be able to 'walk through' the German lines at several places.

That time was now drawing near.

In the battles for Verdun, France was 'bleeding to death' and the British commander, Haig, received frantic appeals to launch an offensive on the Somme to take the pressure off the French. Haig's troops were not ready but he agreed to Joffre's demands. Hospitals got urgent messages to empty as many wards as possible. Long-term wounded were crammed into ambulances and trucks and driven in haste to embarkation ports.

Everyone now knew that the much-talked-about 'big push' that would finish the war was about to be launched. The raw volunteers of Kitchener's army were in the trenches. Very few of them had ever come under fire before or had ever killed a man or even seen death around them. In the pit of their stomachs was a fluttering hollow feeling. Yet the fear of the unknown was buried partly by the novelty and excitement of the occasion. Here they were all gathered together, isolated from the world they had known, where men went to work by day and to the pub with their friends at night. It was a world that other men still enjoyed. Now they were together, dependent on one another. And they were determined to be brave.

Some, no doubt, began to realize what might be in store for them when they were handed the green envelopes into which they could put any private papers they might want to be sent home 'if . . . you know . . .'

By 24 June 1916, the elaborate preparations for the 'big push' were completed. Infantry divisions were packed into front-line positions. There they waited for six days whilst a thunderous Allied artillery barrage exploded onto German wire and trenches. Rain fell heavily during the last two days. At 0730 hours on 1 July, officers blew their whistles. Here finally was the moment for which they had been rehearsing. Infantry clambered up and over the trenches and out into a line, side by side, and advanced at a walking pace as they had so often been drilled.

Suddenly everything seemed to go wrong. The mighty Allied barrage lifted. Even those raw troops knew the shelling should have carried on until the first wave of troops were at least part way across no man's land. Germans raced up from their deep shelters and opened up with machine-guns. The barbed wire was not cut, not 'obliterated' as officers had told them. The half-trained volunteers of Kitchener's army were in real trouble, staggering through the mud, weighed down with sixty-pound packs, ammunition and grenades.

A storm of bullets and mortar shells hit the packed mass of screaming men who were held up on the wire before they even had time to raise their rifles. Wounded huddled in shell-holes. Behind them young subalterns, disdaining the sensible ploy of carrying a rifle so as to be inconspicuous as an officer, came on with their swagger canes. And were felled.

Medical Officer Charles Huxtable noted how those young subalterns had been taught during their brief training to put themselves in front of enemy fire for no other reason than to 'demonstrate leadership'.[3]

It made little difference what anyone was carrying that sunny morning on the Somme. From their strongholds, German gunners could hardly believe their eyes. Never had such easy targets been presented to them. They opened fire. Traversing their guns across the slow-moving lines they knocked down wave after wave in their thousands. Courageously and not knowing what else they could do, young British infantrymen, in hideous confusion, tried to get over or through the wire and hung dead upon it.

The muddy land behind them was strewn with dead. Of the 110,000 men who attacked on that morning, 60,000 were killed or wounded. Never before in the history of warfare had such wanton, pointless carnage been seen in one day. Whole battalions were virtually wiped out. The Newfoundland Regiment, for example, went into the attack 801 strong. When the roll call of the unharmed was taken the next day only sixty-eight answered their names. Every officer was either killed or wounded.

Within three days as the attack continued, casualties approached 100,000. Most commanders would then have called off the offensive, but Haig dare not. To have done so would mean admitting his mistake, so he changed his battle objectives. They were not, he now claimed, to break through German lines and take geographical objectives. Now his aim was to destroy as many Germans as possible, a battle of attrition to wear down the enemy.

If there were those who doubted Haig's new strategy for winning the war then they were unable to convince the War Council, for he survived to carry on his stragegy of attrition on the Somme until mid November 1916.

Some idea of the casualties coming into hospitals can be gained from a picture of a six-acre field behind the lines, covered entirely by stretchers of wounded, lying side by side, waiting to be treated by surgeons or nurses before being taken back to base hospitals.

Yet Haig made little of those casualties. His reports to the press expressed satisfaction that 'we got our first thrust home and there is every reason to be sanguine as to the result'. Stretcher-bearers and nurses were far from sanguine.

Attempts to locate wounded men between the lines and to bring them back to safety became a nightmare. Shelling had pitted the battlefield heavily with craters, which filled up with rainwater, making the whole area a quagmire. By the time the wounded got back to nursing care in hospital they were in a horrendous state and there was never enough time for appropriate treatment. Serving in the 13th Stationary Hospital then was Major Nuttall. He explained that there was never enough time to deal properly with patients, even though a man's chances of survival depended mainly upon the amount of time a doctor or nurse could give him. Blood transfusions were not then a common procedure but when Major Nuttall witnessed the benefits of them he was quite taken aback. The soldier who was on his deathbed beforehand sat up shortly afterwards and asked for a cigarette.[4]

Sister Elsie Grey served in a special hospital for those suffering from head injuries. Often surgeons and nurses would have to work continuously when the wounded poured into the hospital:

> It was simply ghastly. They were all operated on and we never stopped day or night for four or five days. It is terrible to see them wounded in the head – numbers of them became paralysed and quite a number were minus arms or legs or eyes. For the first few days they were quite silly – lost their reason or quite speechless. Oh it was ghastly and very busy – we just went on and on doing dressings with no hope of finishing. The orderlies and padres were awfully good in the wards – taking the men drinks and so forth. I don't know what we would have done sometimes without them. An awful lot of them died of course. We worked hard in the daytime and oh, the nights were terrible. Matron put ten of us out to sleep in two large marquees. We didn't like it of course but we had to pick up our camp beds and get into them like lambs.[5]

Those nurses did not like being under canvas; they felt so vulnerable to shell attack with no protective building overhead.

> I will never forget the first night as long as I live. I woke up suddenly, sat up in bed and then realised what was happening – the Hun aeroplane was directly overhead and the anti-aircraft and machine guns were thundering up at it with terrible force. Oh, it was terrifying – the shrapnel falling in all directions – first on the trees knocking off the boughs at the side of our tent, then on the tent itself. The bullets were whizzing through the air and sounding like dozens of dogs howling and the flashes were reflected into our tent. I was speechless with terror.

Many hospitals then were sufficiently far behind the lines to be out of range or artillery fire, but there were others sited far too close to the front line for comfort. A letter from the hospital matron of one such hospital tells of the death of a very young nursing sister. 'The child was asleep in bed when she was hit. I got to her side in about three minutes. She only knew me for a moment and then mercifully became unconscious and remained so until she passed away fifteen minutes later.'[6]

Another hospital was sited close to a bridge, over a well-used railway line and in front of a heavy artillery battery: all attractive targets for German gunners. Nursing sisters had a very difficult time dealing with a stream of casualties by day when shells were falling on the railway line and being unable to sleep at night due to the cannonade of British artillery. After two weeks of torment by day and night the hospital colonel evacuated the hospital to the lane between some high banks known as the Sunken Road, but while he was supervising the move he was wounded and became another casualty for the nurses to tend.

Elsie Grey's diary records what happened to some of those nurses on that section of the front line.

She described how eighty-nine of them had turned up after being shelled out of neighbouring casualty clearing stations. An English nurse died when some shrapnel came through the tent canvas and entered her sub-clavicle artery. Other fatalities of the shelling included three orderlies. A Canadian sister had lost an eye. As soon as those surviving nursing sisters reached Elsie Grey's hospital they lay down on the floor exhausted and fell asleep straight away. The effects of shell-shock were to take their toll on many of those sisters.[7]

'Battle fatigue', 'disturbed neurosis' or 'shell-shock' (now known as Post-traumatic Stress Disorder, or PTSD) were diagnoses now creeping ever more frequently on to the casualty lists. Soldiers who had steadfastly served for over two years in the trenches meeting horrors anew eventually could take no more. 'It's hard to put the feelings into words but there is a limit to what you can stand seeing day after day, arms and legs blown away from bodies, faces burnt beyond recognition so that you can no longer recognize even your best friend. Your whole being shies away from it like a frightened horse and whatever you do you just can't force yourself to go back into the noise of shelling and machine-gunning,' said Harold Bickerstaff.[8] He was lucky, though many who saw him in fits of coughing from gas-damaged lungs for the rest of his life might not have thought so. A simple gash in his leg from barbed wire turned septic and he was evacuated with blood poisoning.

Sadly Harry Farr, who had volunteered for the army before the war and served with the West Yorkshire Regiment in the trenches for two years, including the Somme battles, was less fortunate. He had been evacuated to hospital suffering from such bad shell-shock that a nurse had to write his letters home to his wife because his hand shook so much.

Eventually he recovered sufficiently to rejoin his battalion in the front line, but his nerves were too far gone and for the next few months he was in and out of hospital. When he was discharged from hospital on the last occasion he could not face returning to the trenches. He refused.

On 2 October 1916 he was put before a court martial. No officer was detailed to conduct his defence, so he told the court himself that he was just no longer fit enough to face gunfire. His sergeant-major had responded to his refusal by shouting back that he would 'blow my fucking brains out himself if I didn't go'.

His company commander told the court that Private Farr's character and conduct were very good except when under fire. Then he was incapable of keeping his head and likely to cause the rest of the men to panic. Farr's platoon commander gave evidence to the effect that when on working parties Farr was trembling and not in a fit state.[9]

The trial for Harry Farr's life lasted twenty minutes. Three senior officers, knowing the pressure put upon them from above, quickly found Farr guilty of showing cowardice in front of the enemy. The sentence, guilty; the punishment, death.

He was tied to a firing post and shot at 6 o' clock on the morning of 18 October 1916 by a firing squad of men from his own regiment who had been fighting alongside him for months.

The wife of Private Harry Farr received a letter frm the War Office. It read:

Dear Madam,
    We regret to inform you that your husband has died. He was sentenced for cowardice and shot at dawn on 18th October.

Her pension was stopped.

But court martials could not cure the condition of shell-shock. Towards the end of the war, more men than ever before, on both sides, were suffering from what was later termed 'disturbed neurosis'. Over 3,000 men of the British army were charged and sentenced to death. Of these, 300 were shot at dawn, and the remainder had their sentences commuted to imprisonment.

Pressure was put on regimental medical officers not to send men back to hospital with a breakdown of nerve or shell-shock. Decisions had to be reached and mistakes were made in the process. Captain Huxtable, a regimental medical officer, admitted having pangs of remorse about not invaliding a soldier back to base for fear of having to deal with a flood of similar cases later. He never forgot the situation of an officer who reported sick having stuck an indelible pencil in his eye just before the battle of the Somme. The pencil's mark was obvious on the white of the eye, which looked inflamed, but Huxtable did not think he ought to excuse the man from taking part in the attack the next morning. The man perished in that attack. Such events preyed on Nuttall's mind subsequently despite the fact that he felt he made the best decision he could on each occasion.[10]

On another occasion, though, nurses in a casualty clearing station brought an officer to him who was on his way back up the line after having lost an eye in a bomb accident some months previously. Gallantly he had volunteered to go back to his unit in the front line. He was a brave man who really did not need to prove anything. Huxtable walked with him up the support trench to the front, but every time one of the guns went off he would fall to the ground trembling. He insisted on going on but when they got to the officer's unit, Huxtable spoke to the commanding officer and suggested the officer be sent back as soon as possible. Having lost an eye he had lost his nerve with it.

Nurses did their best to make the wounded as comfortable as possible for their journey back to base hospitals. At the 13th Stationary Hospital at Boulogne nurses had another job which kept some of them permanently occupied. They had to make sure that every wounded man was given a tetanus anti-toxin and a typhoid vaccine. But it was almost impossible to keep abreast of the treatment needed by casualties streaming into the care of the nurses. Nurse Doris Neve in a recent BBC interview still remembered how the ambulance service carried the wounded into the ward and just put them on to beds still in their muddy clothes, and how one of those soldiers still had the strength to take a gold watch from his pocket, and say, 'Give this to my son,' before dying.[11]

Soldiers whose wounds were not so serious went into a different ward. Their progress was evident in the way they soon began to flirt with the nurses, as Doris remembered some fifty years later how she and her young colleagues would go into the soldiers' wards at night to talk to them and cheer them up. They had to take care to avoid the matron or night sister but thought it was worth the risk as the men eagerly anticipated their clandestine visits.

Norah Clay spoke about the way nurses developed this feeling of wanting to care for their patients, something which she referred to as 'motherliness'. Despite the fact that they were only just into their twenties they felt accountable for the injured soldiers' progress because they had looked after them so personally.[12]

To nurses the Somme battle seemed to be the height of criminal stupidity, as Beryl Hutchinson, a first aid nursing yeomanry driver bringing casualties to hospital wrote in a letter home that the terror of the preceding thirteen days could not have been envisaged even by a 'raving lunatic'.[13]

By November 1916 the fighting on the Somme had degenerated into a series of savage attacks and counter-attacks until both sides were too debilitated to continue.

British losses totalled 420,000 and the French had lost 204,000. Joffre, the French commander-in-chief, lost his job, while his British equivalent, Haig, was promoted to field marshal in January 1917 and survived to lose another 300,000 men in the battle of Passchendaele.

During the last weeks of 1916 murmurings about peace began to be heard on both sides. General Ludendorf no longer boasted of a total victory for Germany. His army had lost 670,000 men in the Somme battles and that superbly trained and equipped German army was no more. After the Somme it had to rely upon youthful levies just as raw as those reinforcing British and French armies. Another source of anxiety, too, for the Germans towards the end of the Somme battles were British tanks, which could push their way through barbed wire and across trenches.

In twenty-one months of war French casualties amounted to more than three million men. In the last days of April 1917, disaster struck. French troops mutinied against incompetent leadership, leaving only two reliable divisions between Paris and the Germans.

Few British nurses heard anything of the French mutiny nor of mutineers shot or thousands banished to Devil's Island and penal battalions in North Africa. They were always busy. At 59th British Hospital at Amiens, Elsie Grey recalled that: 'It was simply ghastly how the wounded poured in. We just went on and on with no hope of finishing. The hospital suffered air attacks. Two casualty clearing stations at Bailliout were evacuated following direct shellfire which killed 70 patients and four nursing sisters.'[14]

Albina Pinninger looked after the wounded from the Somme and Passchendaele battles. 'It was one of the coldest winters ever and the casualties came pouring in, wounded and half frozen. Sometimes we worked in a château near the fighting line. The floor was covered with straw and the ground trembled with the vibration of the guns.'

Then when the manpower situation was getting desperate medical officers and nursing sisters were told that their efforts should be directed mainly towards officers and other ranks who were *lightly* wounded, because they could recover quickly and get back to their depleted units – units that could ill-afford the loss of experienced soldiers. Every experienced man could make a big difference to morale and efficiency.

The aim of most hospitals in France was to get patients back to their units as quickly as possible, or else to get the long-term wounded on to the evacuation trains to Britain so as to free beds for emergencies. Unfortunately the hospital trains often ran the risk of being attacked from the air by German pilots, who regarded all trains, whether bearing the Red Cross emblems or not, as legitimate targets. Many unit war diaries carried references to windows being shattered and woodwork splintered. For journeys at night no lights were allowed, but even so hospital trains were bombed. Wounded men gained strength from seeing the unruffled way sisters carried on regardless of bombs bursting alongside the track.

The final stage of a casualty's journey back to 'Blighty' began with the arrival of a hospital train at the port of embarkation, either in the Middle East or in northern France. Hospital ships plying across the Channel often did two journeys a day during the time of heavy offensive operations, such as those of 1916 and 1917. Then nursing sisters coped by keeping to a well-tried routine.

Before one patient was taken aboard sisters made sure that their own wards had beds ready, as well as meals, warm water-bottles and facilities prepared for those who were going to be sea-sick – as many were. But there were far worse hazards to be faced, as Sister Essington-Nelson found. She was on her way home on a hospital ship, as she later wrote in her diary: 'It was after a battle which finally finished me off. Forty-five terrible cases were brought into my ward. Fifteen died before morning and as a Catholic I went to see each of them and prayed as he died.'

She was grateful to her matron for granting home leave and was to sail on the hospital ship *Anglia*, a former Mail steamer. It had loaded its full complement of patients, when it glided silently out of Boulogne harbour on 17 November 1915. On board were 400 patients, with three nursing sisters and a matron to look after them. Essington-Nelson was helping in a large ward aft whilst Sister Walton was responsible for the two centre wards, in which lay fifty-six cot cases so badly wounded that none of them could move.

Sister Walton went to get some pain-killing tablets from the drugs chest on deck and was there when a large explosion tore into the

centre of the ship. The horrific scene was indelibly printed on
Essington-Nelson's mind:

Sister Walton found herself standing on a sterilizer with her legs
tightly pinned with masses of twisted iron from cots and water
swirling in and out as the ship swayed from side to side amongst the
most awful groans.

She realised that all 50 of the patients below had gone in the blast
from the bomb and eight officers around her were drowning before
her eyes. She, pinned and powerless, could not move. She just
prayed. Another awful explosion shook the boat and she felt herself
being freed but with water now above her head. All she could see
was a faint light above her where the companionway once was. She
was a good swimmer and swam towards the light. She surfaced near
a cupboard for life jackets. She shouted for help and a medical
orderly heard and came running. He opened the cupboard.

Essington-Nelson saw that the deck was covered with wounded
men. Along with medical orderlies, she set about tying them into life
jackets and dropped them into the sea.

We made sure that all splints on legs were removed first otherwise
once in the sea the wooden splints would rise to the surface bringing the legs with them and perhaps make the head go under. Nearly
three hundred men were saved. I saw one wounded man near the
edge of the ship but he just could not lift himself over. Quickly I
took off my own life belt and tied it onto him and pushed him over-
board too. Sister Walton now near to me stood and made her act of
contrition and prayed. She said she felt happy and had no fear. Then
two burly stokers took hold of her and said 'We're not going to let
you drown.' They picked her up and threw her into the arms of a
sailor on a destroyer which had just drawn alongside.[15]

Reports of the incident say there was no panic whatsoever and that
patients and nurses kept their heads wonderfully well. It was only
when the ship's stern rose high in the water, with both propellers
spinning furiously, that nurses and orderlies abandoned further efforts
at rescue. Those nurses and crew left on board then jumped into the
sea.

Hundreds now were struggling to keep afloat. Some in their
desperation clung to one side of a lifeboat, which then capsized, fling-
ing its occupants into the water. Most of those wearing life jackets

were picked up by a destroyer and given warm clothes from officers and crew. They were given a good meal, and by the time they reached Dover all except the wounded were ready to make the train journey to London.

For British and French soldiers on the Western Front in 1917, it looked as though their fortunes were about to turn dramatically for the better. A new beginning came when the liner *Laconia*, carrying American nationals, was torpedoed without warning. To make the Americans more antagonistic towards Germany, two more American ships were sunk – the *City of Memphis* and *Illinois*, with further loss of lives. President Wilson called a special session of Congress and a state of war between the United States and Germany was declared. Soon, thousands of fresh American soldiers would be fighting alongside the war weary ones of the Allies.

British nurses throughout all hospitals toasted the Americans with local wine. Here indeed was hope for the end of the war. They were not aware then how small was the United States regular army, which comprised only 77,000 men with equipment bordering on obsolete. The Americans also had only fifty-five aircraft, fit for nothing more than reconnaissance. Nonetheless, everyone had faith that soon the country would raise a mighty force. With compulsory military service for all able-bodied males between the ages of eighteen and forty-five the army would very soon be coming to the aid of the Allies.

It was not long before a few young nurses were breaking all the hospital rules as they marched up and down the wards singing:

> Over there. Over there.
> Send the word, send the word. Over there.
> That the Yanks are coming
> The Yanks are coming
> There's a drum drum drumming over there.

For General Ludendorff there was no time to lose. He would have to make his last big attack before those Yanks did indeed arrive. And so he did.

# 11 Year of Decision

When this blessed war is over
Oh how happy I shall be
When I get my civvy clothes on
No more soldiering for me.

Tommy Atkins sang it with feeling to the tune of a well-known hymn. The youthful exuberance of those Yanks singing 'The Yanks are coming' did not communicate itself to the French *poilu* or British Tommy. By the end of 1917 their one-time songs of confident warriors had changed to those of soldiers sickened by it all, typified in the various versions of the 'blessed war' song and what they could do with the sergeant-major and his pace stick.

The same spirit was seen by nurses in hospital wards. Soldiers recovering from their wounds no longer wanted to go back to their units 'to have another bash at the Hun', as some had boldly declared in the early days of the war. More often than not by 1918, they were ready to do anything to prolong their convalescence, sometimes even pleading with doctors for a 'Blighty' category that would put them on the boat home. Those who did go back to their units in the line found that things were changing for everyone, nurses and soldiers alike. March 1918 marked the beginning of a new phase of activity altogether. Static trench warfare ended suddenly. And with that came the need for greater mobility of casualty clearing stations and hospitals. Nurses became expert in packing and moving at short notice.

Out of the morning mists of Saint-Quentin on 21 March 1918 three German armies launched an offensive with a barrage of poison gas and high-explosive shells fired from 6,500 guns. After the barrage came an attack led by special storm troops reinforced by experienced soldiers from the Eastern Front. They broke the British line, leaving the fortified redoubts for others to clear later.

Nurses in hospitals anywhere near this front were confronted with the problem of caring for an enormous number of new casualties – 165,000 of them British – and at the same time preparing to pack and move at a moment's notice. This situation was vividly depicted in a letter home from a Territorial Army nursing sister who wrote:

> One morning we were called at five o'clock and told to put our gas masks onto the alert position as gas shells were coming over. We had a hurried breakfast and then the wounded started to come in. I had a ward full of patients for resuscitation, penetrating wounds of the abdomen, chests, heads, and cases requiring immediate amputation of limbs. Medical officers, non-commissioned officers and nurses just worked at high pressure as long as we could. All the time we had to work with our gas-masks at the Alert but I hung mine on my back.[1]

Early in the afternoon the hospital's commanding officer sent an urgent message to all wards to clear out at once. They filled the ambulances with the worst cases and some sisters went in each one. When they were on the road to the next casualty clearing station they came under fire, but most of the shells dropped in the fields along-side. No one was hurt. Nurses were less concerned for their own safety than that of their patients, some of whom had just come out of the operating theatre.

They had just stopped at the site of another casualty clearing station and were about to unpack when orders came for them to move everyone to the nearby railway station as quickly as possible. German infantry were close at hand. Once there they waited over an hour for the hospital train; shells rained down all around them.

With the enemy barely twenty minutes away the train arrived and everyone got away to Number 50 CCS, where nurses immediately started attending patients again. 'The first day I fed the operating theatres and kept the tables going with dressings and gloves. Men seemed just to pour in. Surgeons and the Matron were simply splendid. They worked with the rest of the staff day and night. There was no time for regular meals or sleep,'[2] recalled Sister G. Wicker.

Women of the First Aid Nursing Yeomanry (FANY) ambulance unit brought casualties from the front to the casualty clearing station. They had crossed to France in 1914 with their own motorized ambulances, and disregarding the hostility of some who still did not like the idea of women in what was traditionally a man's world, they soon distinguished themselves by the way they continued to drive their ambulances down roads, under shell fire or not. They took a pride in getting the wounded back.

When Ludendorf launched his attack on 21 March, sections of the FANY ambulance corps, based in Amiens, read with anxiety Haig's order of the day, published when the Allies were in full retreat: 'With our backs to the wall and believing in the justice of our cause, each one of us must fight to the end.'

FANY drivers immediately began a round-the-clock shuttle service taking wounded from hospitals to trains heading for Channel ports. As drivers lifted the wounded into the ambulances, they noticed an odd smell that caught in their throats causing them to cough. Gas. From men on stretchers waiting to be loaded came the sound of painful, almost continuous hacking. Some of these men had their eyes tightly closed with tears of pain squeezing out from under their reddened lids. Their rasping, agonized breathing together with the bluish tinge of their lips showed just how much damage had already been done to their lung tissues.

Ambulances pulled in to casualty clearing stations hastily set up in village halls and schools. Stretchers littered floors from wall to wall. 'The whole place seemed to vibrate with the tension brought on by an awareness of death in an atmosphere reeking with the stench of blood and cordite, and sweat. Added to all that was the sound of crying and groaning as nurses rushed about everywhere and doctors worked doggedly over serried rows of stretchers,' wrote Madge Swann in her diary. 'Occasionally I had to wait alongside a nursing sister putting a new dressing on a patient before sending him off in the ambulance and I could hardly bear to look at the mess of flesh and bone splinters that once were part of a leg or arm.'[3]

Mustard gas burns presented a problem for nurses. Various dressings were tried, but eventually one of the favourites was a dressing produced by Boot's the Chemist and advertised thus in the *Journal of Nursing*:

Spray with Chlorocosane solution of dichloramine-T 5%. Then apply to burns melted Number 7 Paraffin Wax with a large camel hair brush to form a wax glazing. On this quickly place a thin layer of cotton wool. Afterwards cover the cotton wool with more melted Number 7 Paraffin Wax to ensure an air tight dressing. This should be renewed every twenty-four hours. Later it can be left for forty-eight hours.

While nurses were still caring for patients the retreat went on, but soon there was no transport for the 'walking wounded'. They just had to totter and stumble alongside the railway track. Men with arm wounds acted as crutches for men wounded in the leg – a pathetic sight.

During the whole of the period of retreat, when nurses were in great danger, Dame Maud McCarthy was on the move ceaselessly, visiting casualty clearing stations and talking to QA nurses and VADs. She made detailed notes about what was needed and how conditions might be improved, noting the deaths and injuries among them and what the consequent staffing arrangements could be for casualty clearing stations and hospitals.

In one of her reports to the director general of Army Medical Services she commended all nurses for the way they had got on with their jobs in a 'businesslike and orderly manner' while battles raged close by. She told how in one air raid when four nurses were crossing a railway line a bomb killed one of them and severely wounded another. One nurse stayed behind, caring for the wounded nurse while the fourth nurse ran to the nearest casualty clearing station for help. A little later that evening those same two QAs went on duty in the operating theatre all night, 'displaying the most wonderful courage'. Both nursing sisters were awarded the Military Medal.

In another report Dame Maud McCarthy also noted how highly she regarded the service of the VADs. They had very little training compared with the fully trained QA personnel. In one report she wrote:

Anyone who has seen the trained and the untrained nurses working together during the weeks following the recent battles would have realized that any feeling of resentment there once might have been was only of a superficial character, and that each was only too anxious to help the other, so that they might the better devote themselves to the service of the sick and the wounded.

Within eight days German troops had advanced forty miles, and by 27 May they had reached the Marne at Château-Thierry, from which they had been driven four years earlier, thirty-seven miles from Paris. Now thousands of demoralized French soldiers threw away their rifles and uniforms and vanished into civilian crowds streaming along roads towards Paris.

Fortunately by this time the forward units of the German army were also suffering from exhaustion and insufficient supplies. The fighting tapered off. The Allies consolidated their defensive positions and the Germans prepared to attack on another front.

Paris was safe. Or was it?

An unexpected new development brought further anxiety to Parisians and nurses in Paris hospitals in that third week of March 1918. A massive explosion shook buildings and broke windows over a wide area. Twenty minutes later, before the populace had time to work out what had caused such a thunderous detonation, another explosion killed eight citizens and seriously wounded thirteen others.

A hurried examination of fragments of metal close to the scene of the explosions established the fact that the jagged chunks came from artillery shells. Paris was being shelled by new top-secret guns with a range of seventy-five miles.

One of the most tragic effects from shots fired by those guns happened at 4.30 one afternoon when one of their huge high-explosive shells landed among the kneeling worshippers packed into the church of Saint-Gervais in the centre of Paris. Tons of masonry cascaded upon the congregation, killing eighty-eight of them and critically injuring a further sixty-eight.

The morale of civilians and soldiers had never been lower.

There then began a second 'reign of terror' in Paris, as the new German big guns poured 370 shells into the French capital, making no distinction between hospitals, houses or factories. This new setback, coming in the wake of the defeatism and mutinies amongst French units, alerted the government to the hazards of tottering morale. Gangs of builders were rushed to each Paris area wrecked by the new shelling to remove all debris and repair buildings straight away.

It was not only from the big guns that Paris and the British nurses in hospitals there suffered, they had to bear the brunt of new attacks from bomber aircraft. These became so desperate as to be almost suicidal as far as the pilots were concerned. They refused to be deviated from their targets no matter how fierce the anti-aircraft fire and attacks from patrolling Allied fighter planes might be.

Air raids became part of a last desperate German attempt to wear down Allied resolution. Four QA nursing sisters were killed in the hospital at Saint-Omer during an air raid. While evacuating casualties, ambulances were often attacked from the air. It was a hazard constantly faced by young drivers of the Women's Transport Service. In May 1918, they were taking casualties from a raid on an ammunition dump that lasted three hours. Such was the courage and devotion to duty shown by those women that sixteen Military Medals and two Croix de Guerre were awarded to the drivers of the FANY ambulances and their VAD crews.

While German manpower shortage was now critical, Allied armies were being reinforced by newly arrived, though inexperienced, American troops. On 28 May the American 1st Division routed the Germans in a brief but furious battle. Then on 6 June 1918, Marines of the American 2nd Division attacked and cleared German infantry from the highly fortified Belleau Wood. In doing so the division suffered 9,777 casualties.

On 15 July the American 2nd Division attacked the dumbfounded Germans assaulting Allied positions on the Marne. Bloody hand-to-hand combat stopped the Germans in their tracks.

Beryl Hutchinson was very busy with her ambulance unit of the First Aid Nursing Yeomanry along the River Marne that summer of 1918. The procedure was for casualties arriving from the front to be sorted into categories – those who could withstand a bumpy journey by motor ambulance under shellfire, to hospital ships and the more serious cases who would benefit from the gentler journey to the coast in well-equipped hospital barges.[4]

Once again Allied nurses were stretched to the limit, looking after enormous numbers of casualties. To give a comprehensive account of their service in these latter months of the war would be impossible without telling and retelling similar experiences. Nevertheless the selection of a few more personal accounts here will help to show the many ways in which nurses in France and Germany contributed to victory. They had, of course, already done so by their service in many different parts of the world and in many different nursing capacities.

The experience of so many nurses was expressed by Sister Sybil Harry in a letter to her former matron, Miss Cooke. She told how horrific were the wounds caused by the new German artillery guns. Not only were the injuries horrendously big but the wounds soon turned septic and nothing much could be done for these patients. She felt that it was heartless not to allow them to 'sleep their lives away'. She also wrote about how a bullet lodged in the body often caused a large abscess. A major operation was required and this, in most cases, resulted in death. She was also taken aback at how many of her patients developed tetanus and that almost two-thirds of them died a terrible death shortly afterwards.[5]

Sister Mayne at that time lived through what she described as 'a nightmare of suffering':

When every nurse and doctor was on duty going from stretcher to stretcher and bed to bed, we just had to get our priorities right cleaning wounds, applying dressings, giving morphine, and saline for shock and drinks. Then onto the next poor lad.

We got water from the pump in the yard and we heated it on the
coke stove in the centre of the ward. There were so many men lying
there that it was difficult to get around yet in spite of everything a
certain cheerfulness pervaded all.[6]

So short of men were British divisions after four gruelling years of
war that back home men were being taken from previously reserved
occupations, and the age limit for compulsory military service was
raised to fifty. Nurses were affected by this critical manpower shortage. Again and again they were given 'guidance' as to the time to be
spent on wounded soldiers. Their time and skill was to be directed
more towards the recovery of lightly wounded men, so that they
could be posted back to their units in the line as quickly as possible.
The message given to them earlier was emphasized. Time spent in
getting lightly wounded men back to the fighting line was more
productive than time spent on seriously wounded men that would
never fight again. Sister Mary Sybil Towers, who listened to this guidance from her medical officer, recalled: 'It was hard saying that to us
Sisters, but I knew what he meant, and did not misunderstand him.'

Fortunately by then, though none of the nurses realized it, the tide
of war had turned for the last time. At precisely 4.20 a.m. on 8
August 1918, British, French, Australian, Canadian and American
divisions were about to launch their final attack. The Americans
brought 600 of their latest tanks. Ahead of them was a mess of craters
and hummocks bounded by formidable lines of tangled barbed wire
peopled only by the decomposing bodies of soldiers from both sides
who had taken part in earlier offensives.

Now the attackers had to endure an awful waiting period. This
time the offensive was to be different. With tanks in the lead and
bomber aircraft overhead, the infantry advanced at a run behind a
creeping barrage from 2,000 guns. This time there was no walking
together in line.

Troops were assembled with such secrecy that when the attack
went in one German division was taken so much by surprise that they
were caught in the middle of eating lunch! Behind an intense artillery
barrage Allied infantry advanced, their ears battered by the sound and
vibrating pressure of the air. Even the ground beneath their feet
seemed to shudder. Steadily they moved forward, the speed of their
advance determined by the moving curtain of shells. If the men
moved too quickly they would run into bursting shells from their own
guns. By nightfall leading battalions were nine miles behind the
German front line.

The German infantry was demoralized. So too was their commander-in-chief, General Erich Ludendorff. In his diary he wrote: 'August
8th was the black day of the German Army. Morale was no longer
what it had been.'

No longer was the General scornful of the Americans.

The end was obviously near on 8 September, when a massive force
of 550,000 Americans and 110,000 French attacked near Metz. A day
and a half later 16,000 German prisoners, 450 guns and 400 square
miles had been taken. American divisions suffered 7,000 casualties.

Now nurses in hospitals and casualty clearing stations were moving
forward more quickly than ever before, and they paid little attention
to the intermittent shelling to which all approach routes were
subjected.

In that late summer of 1918, once casualties reached hospitals in
Britain, their wounds began to be dressed by a new method which
nurses found less painful for the patient and avoided future dressings
sticking to the wound. The method was used by Sir Almroth Wright
at St Mary's Hospital, Paddington. It involved putting a thin piece of
perforated celluloid on the wound before the dressing went on. The
celluloid was soaked first in a carbolic acid solution and then rinsed in
a weak salt solution. This soft film of celluloid was put gently on to
the wound followed by the fine lint and bandages. The hospital no
longer used antiseptics for such wounds. A report in the *British
Journal of Nursing* concluded 'The surgeon in charge says that the
wounds are kept wet with a weak salt and water solution and that is
all the local treatment they get.'[7]

Surgeons were trying other new ways of repairing some of the
terribly mutilated bodies. A journalist visiting one of London's military hospitals spoke with a surgeon who was trying to help a soldier
with a shattered arm. Repair was going to be difficult, however,
because four inches of a nerve had been destroyed. The surgeon tele-
phoned around London hospitals to enquire if any arm amputations
were to take place. Finding one about to be amputated that very
afternoon, he asked for it to be placed in a saline bath and brought to
him straight away in a taxi. Placing his own patient under anaesthetic
he dissected from the amputated limb the four inches of nerve and
grafted it into the severed nerve of the patient. The result was
successful.[8]

The removal of a piece of shrapnel embedded in the muscle of a
heart was another triumph of modern surgery demonstrated that day.

Severe facial disfigurement was another problem for surgeons to
deal with when patients got back to London. Many were not only

scarred beyond recognition, but to such an extent that young children ran away in terror from their returning fathers, with part of a cheek bone or eye missing.

So great was the problem that a special surgical hospital with a hundred beds was set up at Sidcup, to cope with the stream of burnt and shattered faces. New techniques of plastic surgery were pioneered there, and for those who had insufficient skin and tissue left to take grafts, masks were made – 'tin faces' – to hide gross disfigurement.

It was at Sidcup between 1917 and 1925 that Archibald McIndoe, renowned for his treatment of RAF aircrew at East Grinstead in World War Two, worked as an assistant to plastic surgeon Harold Gillies.

In the early ears of the First World War casualties with severe facial injuries were given a low priority, and many of them died from shock, to which they were understandably prone.

When some patients realized that no one could look upon them, even their loved ones, without feelings of revulsion, they lost all will to live and just died. Others took even more drastic steps and killed themselves, so as not to be a lifetime burden on their wives and families. The standard procedure followed by hospitals for suicides in such cases was a telegram to next of kin with this short message:

The War Office regrets to inform you that your son, Corporal Thomas A —— of the Manchester Regiment died this morning after a relapse.

Patients gained more hope after treatment at Sidcup. Harold Gillies believed in starting procedures as soon as possible. Consequently the recovery rate of patients improved enormously.

The first stage of their recovery, though, was in the hands of nurses and doctors in casualty clearing stations and field hospitals. They were responsible for cleaning up the awesome facial holes where bones and flesh had been blasted away so that some healing could begin prior to reconstructive surgery later.

When there was not enough tissue and bone left for plastic surgery to be practicable, the long process of mask-making began. Molds were made, starting with ones built up from plaster-of-Paris casts. The inner surface of the casts replicated the mutilated holes in the face, which had now healed sufficiently for work to begin. The outer surface could then be sculpted to match whatever was left or to match as near as possible the shape and likeness of the soldier's face taken from photographs before being disfigured.

Eye sockets were difficult, but sculptors working with scrupulous artistry shaped the eyebrow and socket to blend inconspicuously with the rest of the face.

As the summer of 1918 merged into autumn the fruits of a series of Allied summer offensives began to be seen. Britain, France and the United States had planned for another year of war but they were now fighting against a German army afflicted with a feeling of hopelessness. Morale throughout all ranks was at its lowest point. Allied losses had now been replaced by 600,000 fresh troops from the United States, which took the field in force under General Pershing. They had distinguished themselves already at Château-Thierry, and now with hundreds of light mobile tanks they were able to pierce German defences.

Suddenly an astonishing succession of Allied victories brought German resistance to breaking-point. First Bulgaria, then Turkey, then Austria were so emphatically defeated that they sued for peace. For a few weeks the German army, badly shaken, carried on fighting but German civilians, hungry and miserable, wanted peace.

Finally Ludendorff's nerve broke. At a routine German staff meeting he ranted hysterically, blaming everyone but himself. He wept and toppled to the floor in nervous prostration. That night he advised Hindenburg to sue for peace. On 9 November Hindenburg warned the Kaiser that the German army was now powerless to protect him, adding, 'I must advise Your Majesty to abdicate and proceed to Holland.'

General Pershing pressed his political masters to pursue the war to complete victory and unconditional surrender. His proposals were ignored. Somehow, German generals withdrew into the shadows and took no part in the armistice proceedings, which were conducted by the civil government.

Ludendorff, disguised with dark glasses and a civilian suit, slipped quietly into neutral Sweden. Then, insidiously but surely, the German generals spread the propaganda that it had never been defeated, just 'stabbed in the back' by political traitors at home.

German soldiers who had fought those final battles never for a moment doubted that they had been soundly beaten. Lieutenant Otto Strasser had been with the 4th German Artillery Regiment from August 1914 until the end in 1918, and later emerged as leader of the Black Front opposition to Hitler. Recovering from a heart attack in his sick bed at the Benedictine hospital, Tutzing, he explained to me just how awful it was for German infantry in autumn 1918:

No German soldier who had fought in those last few battles and seen the contrast between the starved, ragged and exhausted figures of our diminishing army, and the well-nourished, splendidly equipped, well-trained and well-rested lads of the innumerable American armies, can ever believe in the stupid and venomous fairy-tale of the 'Stab-in-the-back'.

Our divisions were no stronger than a single regiment. Reinforcements were made up of half-grown lads and fifty-year-olds, fathers, grandfathers, sick and half-invalided men. Their boots were of odd bits of leather held together by cobbler's thread. The spirit was one of desperation. Murmurs of mutiny were in the air. Our troops were inferior. The game was up.

Nevertheless, Germans under the rising star of Hitler came to believe they had never been beaten in the field. And three years after the armistice was signed two former German officers shot and killed the man who signed the Armistice, Erzberger, as a 'traitor'.

So it was that twenty-one years after 'the war to end all wars' finished, the Allies were having to go to war again. This time, though, the aim was definitely different. This time Germany would have to be beaten and to surrender unconditionally to the supreme Allied commander.

In the years between the two world wars, middle-aged men and women would emerge stiffly out of coaches to view the countryside around Delville Wood or Thiepval and think the place looked just as dull as it did before. Yet there would come to them the ghosts of pals they had lost, and snatches of songs, and they would smell the poppies and moonpennies along the roads they had plodded on their way to the trenches, now covered with dandelions and lush clover.

From time to time the coach would stop at cemeteries. Some would walk along the rows, reading the names again on neat head-stones; others were marked simply, 'An Unknown British Soldier'. Soldiers and former nurses alike would pause along the rows of silent graves and remember the courage and the dry, never failing humour of those who had made the ultimate sacrifice. Among those listed on those memorials were the names of 195 nurses.

For those who made journeys of remembrance, memories came unbidden. Memories of trials and sacrifices, poignant and tinged with a sense of the stupid waste of it all, and hopes that surely the same mistakes would never be made again. Yet memories grew dim all too quickly, and threats of another war with Germans loomed larger.

# 12 No Rest for Nurses

'Nothing, save a battle lost, can be half so melancholy as a battle won.'
Duke of Wellington's despatch from the field of Waterloo

The war ended abruptly in the autumn of 1918 taking most nurses, military and civilian, by surprise. One day the newspapers were saying the Allies were on the verge of defeat, yet shortly afterwards their armies were racing into Germany and to an armistice. Could overworked nurses now have a rest?

They could not. The world was still in turmoil. The British army sent divisions to far-off places and nurses went with them, even to that most inhospitable part of the Arctic, the icy, barren north Russian shore of Archangel.

But the more immediate problem for nurses to tackle was the invasion of Britain by an enemy more difficult to fight and even more deadly than German machine-guns and artillery. Its advance could not be checked – an influenza epidemic of the most virulent type hit the country. Already it had taken the lives of 16 million Indians, made its lethal way across the Near East and reached France in the early summer of 1918. Now it was Britain's turn.

Most vulnerable to this new scourge were under-nourished exservicemen with lungs severely damaged by gas. 'Spanish Flu', as it was called, became a pestilence that would kill more men, women and children than four years of warfare.

Poorly clad ex-soldiers could offer little resistance to the virus. Wives and mothers of those former soldiers watched with alarm as their husbands and sons were struck down suddenly with terrible pains in the head, back and legs, with red eyes and a high fever. Doctors said there was nothing to be done except bed rest and the inevitable aspirin. Something like three-quarters of the population of England were struck down.

Good food and rest were the main cure. Some did get better, but many did not. For many did not have good food and rest. Poverty and deprivation were all too common predicaments. The state at that time provided little assistance. Men who applied to the parish for aid were often so humiliated by the parsimonious way money was given out that they never went again. They preferred to remain hungry than have their pride mocked. The houses promised by vote-hunting politicians as 'fit for heroes to live in' never materialized. Terraced slum houses to which soldiers returned were infested with rats and cockroaches and fleas: hot-houses for breeding infection.

Many came home blind, with an arm or leg missing or mentally confused and unable to find regular work. So they begged or sold bootlaces from a tray supported by a strap round their necks. A roughly scrawled notice reminded passers-by who they were: 'DISABLED IN THE WAR'.

At an early age Sister Bessie Strand, then the eldest daughter in a family of four, shouldered the burden of looking after her father, blinded in the war. Even after she left home to work as a nurse she still had that responsibility.[1]

To cope with the human wreckage, nurses were more in demand than ever before. Muriel Palmer, a VAD nurse who had met her husband in France, gave up work to look after him when he returned home in 1918.

He'd been in the Manchester Pals Regiment and was gassed on the Western Front. When he caught a bad dose of the 'flu I sat by his bedside at night and watched him, propped up on pillows, get gradually worse. He sweated so heavily his pyjamas and even the sheets on his bed were soaking wet.

I'd seen too many men desperately ill in France not to recognize the awful signs of a dying man in him; the blueness of his lips, the way his chest caved in at the ribs and the struggle he had to draw breath. I counted each one, as they rasped in and out of his tortured lungs and often in the small hours of the night I would wish that he'd drawn his last one. When he put his hand to his side and grimaced with pain I guessed his 'flu had turned into influenzal pneumonia. The doctor confirmed my fears. We hoped and prayed that having survived the war he would at least recover from this 'flu but with each passing day there was no abatement in his symptoms. We did try warm kaolin poultices to relieve the pain in his side but without much benefit.

The war was over but it then seemed so irrelevant somehow as I sat with him listening to his breathing becoming more erratic and watching him slide out of my fingers. I was murmuring to him about the past in the early hours before dawn one morning when his fingers momentarily clenched mine more firmly. I stopped whispering and looked closely at his face and listened. The struggle to breathe was over. Ever so quietly, my lovely husband left me.[2]

Harold Palmer, late of the Manchester Pals (the official name for the regiment raised from volunteers from that area) was but one of thousands of former soldiers with gas-corrupted lungs who lost their lives during that influenza epidemic. Their deaths were never classed as due to enemy action, however, and no widows' pensions were ever awarded to the wives left behind, often with children to raise.

For German soldiers returning home the situation was even worse in that tempestuous post-war period. Middle-aged men found their lives in ruin about them; young men prematurely old came back from the war and tried to find a way to an ordered family life they had once enjoyed; and confused young lads leaving school wondered how they could possibly find a job and a secure future.

In such a climate of social malaise and economic depression the country was ripe for a dictatorial take-over from left or right. Misery and confusion were not confined to the domestic life of Britain and Germany. The unsettled political order of the post-war world also affected the postings of British servicemen and, of course, their nurses.

In the autumn of 1918, fourteen QAs sailed from Cardiff in the *Kalyan*, a cruise liner converted into a hospital ship for service in Archangel. There they would give medical care to the remnants of the Russian imperial army. In July 1918, four months before the war on the Western Front ended, Allied troops had gone to Russia ostensibly to revive an Eastern Front against the Germans, but with the additional hope that it would help the imperial army to defeat the Bolsheviks. They had overthrown Tsar Nicholas II in the revolution of March 1917 and set up a dictatorship of the proletariat. The British government feared that this might encourage the British Socialist Party. In a convention at Leeds in June 1917 the party called for a British revolution and the setting-up of workers' and soldiers' councils or 'soviets'.

The British government was clearly fearful of the inspirational success of the Russian revolution, and its effect on radicals at home. It was very much in politicians' minds that the Russian revolution had started with a riot in Petrograd on 8 March, a tram strike on the 10th, a regimental mutiny on the 11th and the defection of the household troops on the 12th. The Tsar abdicated on 15 March 1917 and thereafter the whole revolutionary movement spread like a prairie fire. By the end of July 1917, the Russian front had crumbled in face of the German enemy and within weeks the Red revolutionaries surged round the Winter Palace and the Bolsheviks seized power.

The British government, worried that revolutionary ideas might spread to Britain, was more than willing to send a token force with supporting medical services to Archangel, one of the few ice-free ports through which Russian forces loyal to the Tsar could be supplied.

For those fourteen QAs it was no comfortable cruise northwards. Their converted hospital ship had not been fitted for Arctic conditions. Some attempt had been made to keep the passengers warm by lining the ship's hull with wooden walls filled with sawdust, but nurses shivered by day and night as they passed through Arctic darkness, floating ice, blizzards, mountainous seas and such thick fog that the ship's captain hardly dared leave the bridge. The decks, rigging and superstructures were covered with ice, transforming the ship completely.

For all those nurses, that fortnight's voyage was the beginning of an ordeal below zero. Shortly after they arrived at Archangel the ship was frozen in by thick ice. Consequently, the *Kalyan* could no longer operate as a hospital ship, but as a stationary hospital. Nurses were issued with men's warm clothing that comprised sheepskin-lined coats and fur-peaked caps with ear flaps. Casualties were brought from battlelines 200 miles away – sometimes in barges and then, when the river froze, by rail on lines laid over the ice. Some even came in fur-lined sleeping-bags lying on open horse-drawn sleighs.

Understandably, one of the frequent cases needing nurses' attention was frostbite, caused by exposure to extreme cold. After such an episode, arteries in the arm or leg contracted and the limb felt 'dead'. If the limb's exposure to extreme cold was prolonged, it was in danger of becoming gangrenous and requiring amputation. Nurses found the best treatment was to warm the part gently against the body of another soldier, until circulation was restored.

After eight months imprisoned in the harbour by the frozen Arctic Ocean, icebreakers got through and brought with them troopships with relief for nurses and men. It was something of an anti-climax for nurses when the *Kalyan* finally docked in Leith in June 1919. After all, the Great War had been over for seven months, along with the Armistice celebrations – except for the victory parade through London, in which the QAs took part, to great cheers of appreciation from crowds packing the pavements.

Now for the QAIMNS it was time to get down to peace-time nursing and to consolidate their new status. Part of this consolidation was to maintain the link between the civil and military nursing services. This was achieved effectively when Dame Maud McCarthy, who was well remembered for her work in France, was appointed matron-in-chief of the Territorial Auxiliary Nursing Service. The link between military and civilian was strengthened in 1925 when Queen Mary became president of the QAIMNS and of the QAIMNS (Reserves) upon the death of Queen Alexandra.

The following year all QA nursing sisters were granted equivalent rank with the regular army officers. To become a QA nursing sister now was a respectable aim to which young women could aspire. But it was no easy task for them. First of all they had to complete successfully the three basic years of training in a general hospital. Selection boards insisted also on candidates being of pure European descent and having British parents.

During the late 1920s and early 1930s when the QAIMNS grew steadily in prestige and efficiency, nursing sisters were still serving abroad and being posted for many unusual duties. Some had for many years enjoyed serving in the German Rhineland, where in their off-duty hours they could enjoy the amenities of such cities as Cologne, Bonn, Koblenz and Frankfurt. But then apprehension over the possibility of Bolshevism sweeping across a weakened Europe led to the German reoccupation of the Rhineland in 1936 after Adolf Hitler's rise to power.

The Second World War was just three years away.

In those peaceful days of the early 1930s, QAs served abroad in Hong Kong, Gibraltar, Egypt and India but in addition they were on call to help overseas countries suffering natural disasters. On 31 May 1935, for example, QAs were rushed to the town of Quetta, developed by the British in 1876 as a strategic fortress on the north-west frontier of India, controlling the passes into south Afghanistan. The town, standing on hills 5,500 feet high and ringed by other mountains, suddenly shook and crumbled upon itself. Some 60,000 people died and thousands more suffered terrible injuries from falling masonry in the earthquake.

QAs put on a wartime footing served in tented wards and operating theatres. It was a frightening and hazardous experience for all nurses and medical staff. The ground still shook with tremors. Casualties needing more complicated surgery were taken by air to the Mayo hospital at Lahore. This was the first time that casualties were evacuated by air and was a forerunner to the air evacuation services

run by the Royal Navy, Army and Royal Air Force in the Second
World War.

Ironically, one of the last emergency tasks that took QAs abroad
was when the German battleship *Deutschland* was hit by two bombs
off Ibiza during the Spanish Civil War. A hundred German sailors
suffering from burns, complicated by open gashes and fractures, were
cared for by British doctors and nurses at Gibraltar. Severe burns
cases needed special attention and one nurse was allotted to each case
for the first forty-eight hours. For their work with the wounded
sailors, the German Navy awarded the German Red Cross to military
nurses, and afterwards visiting German battleships gave a party with
dancing to which QAs were invited. Everyone had a marvellous time.
The Second World War was now but a mere two years away.

Worries about the fragility of peace were then producing action in
civilian hospitals in the late 1930s. Miss Bishop, matron of Salisbury
Infirmary, called six young and well-qualified nurses into her office
one day. They stood before her with a certain amount of trepidation,
wondering what they had done wrong. After all, this was the matron
who had once sacked all the resident medical staff because they had
gone to a dance without her permission. Those six nurses were not
kept waiting long. Miss Bishop came straight to the point. 'War is
coming,' she said, 'and the Army needs volunteers. You, you, you,
you, you and you will put your names down for the Reserve List right
away.'³ 'Volunteering' British-army style was thenceforth operating.

Meanwhile civilian and service nurses got on with their tiring and
often hazardous jobs. Infection from diseases such as diphtheria, scarlet
fever and typhoid fever, which had very high mortality rates, put nurses
continually at risk from the moment they joined as probationaries.

Freda Barnfather, who later served as a wartime QA in many overseas campaigns, has never forgotten her early days as a probationer
nurse. She was a strong young lady from the north-east with a mind
of her own but tells stories of how life for a young nurse could be
frightening.

I had just left school and was starting my first week of training at
West Goath Hospital and was in a ward when the telephone rang. I
ran in terror to the far end of the ward. I wasn't going to be the one
to answer that call. You see, what frightened me more than anything
was the matron. Well, frightened in some ways but not always. I
remember for example one day just before Christmas when I was
out shopping in London with another probationer nurse. We
suddenly realised we were going to be a few minutes late in getting

back to the hospital. 'Let's run,' said my friend. Typically, I suppose, I said, 'We're going to be late anyway, we might just as well finish our shopping.' So we did.

Next morning, Matron had us both on the carpet. She was such a frosty-faced woman, small and wiry and really nasty. When she thundered a question at me asking why we were late, anger suddenly gave me a rush of courage so I answered in all honesty that we'd been shopping and over-ran the time and then thought that we might as well be hung for a sheep as a lamb. She did not like that at all. But it wasn't an offence for which we could be sent home so we just got a telling off and a warning.[4]

The strict discipline and unappetizing food came as a shock to young probationary nurses and some of them wondered whether they had made the right choice of career. However, many wartime nurses later said that the harsh regime of their training years probably helped them to cope with difficult situations encountered in the war – they just got on with the job. There were rules and a way of doing things.

Late in 1938, qualified nurses who had complied with their matron's 'suggestion' that they should join the QA Reserve were receiving a large envelope through the post. Inside it was another one marked 'TO BE OPENED IN THE EVENT OF WAR'.

They put it away and for the time being forgot about the QA Reserve. That service, however, was well aware of the role it might have to be playing in the not-too-distant future. During the last twenty years it had grown steadily in size and efficiency. The Territorial Army Nursing Service had progressed correspondingly.

By the summer of 1939 war seemed inevitable. At that time there were fewer than 700 regulars in the QAIMNS but under the matron-in-chief, Miss Roy, the QAIMNS Reserve and the Territorial Army Nursing Service were mobilized at speed and welded together into one efficient service.

So it was that during the last week of August 1939, Joan Lister, one of the volunteers for the QA Reserve, received her call-up papers. She opened the sealed envelope and followed its directive. On 1 September 1939 she left Manchester Royal Infirmary bound for the huge military hospital of Netley. The six sisters who 'volunteered' as directed by their matron, Miss Bishop, received their call-up papers about the same time and were given only two hours to pack and report for duty at Netley, too. 'Matron, in her scarlet cape bedecked with medal ribbons met us all briskly, spoke for five minutes and sent us off to buy our uniform in London.'

A day or two later seventy QAs, hastily gathered together at Netley, were equipped with tin hat and gas masks, then hustled aboard a crowded ship at Southampton bound for Cherbourg.

There [recalled Joan] an old soldier met us and gave us some good advice. He told us to go into the town and buy food and drink for a long journey. We bought rolls, sliced sausage meat, apples, cheese and mineral water.

We were certainly thankful for that advice as we sat for hours afterwards on the hard slatted seats of Belgian trains seemingly being shunted up and down tracks going nowhere in the Belgian countryside. Not one of us realised then how long that journey was going to be during the next six years when we were drafted so far and wide in the Second World War.

# 13 Into Battle Again

Our Thirty Corps Casualty Clearing Station was always
located ... well within range of the German guns and the
nurses revelled in it.[1]

Lieutenant General Sir Brian Horrocks

'Grandma is dead!'

Shortly before dawn on 1 September 1939 those three code words
activated German SS men in Polish uniforms to make a bizarre
pretext of an attack on a German radio station at Gleiwitz. To lend
realism to the deception, for reporters to see, concentration camp
prisoners were also dressed in Polish uniforms, given lethal injections
and left on the 'battlefield' as if shot by German defenders. In retal-
iation for the 'attack', German divisions poured across the Polish
frontier. Now there was no way out. Commitments of mutual assistance had been made. On Sunday morning, 3 September, Britain and
France declared war on Germany. That same night at 9 p.m. the
German submarine *U-30* torpedoed and sank the British liner
*Athenia*; 112 passengers lost their lives; twenty-eight were citizens of
the United States. The Second World War had begun .

The next day President Franklin Roosevelt made America's position clear. In a nationwide broadcast he said: 'Let no man or woman
thoughtlessly or falsely talk of America sending its armies to
European fields. At this moment there is being prepared a proclama-
tion of American neutrality.'

So the British public knew where they stood. Alone with France.
Furthermore it was clear that anyone at sea now was likely to be
attacked by U-boats or from the air. Troopships about to carry nurses
and military hospitals to France shortly were particularly vulnerable,
concentrated as they were within the narrow confines of the Channel.
Although the Royal Navy still might claim to rule the waves they did
not rule the air. Consequently troops and nurses did not cross the

149

Channel by the short route from Dover to Calais or Boulogne as they did in 1914, because a thousand German aircraft were poised to pounce on all shipping there.

Within the first few days after the declaration several military hospitals began embarking on troopships at Southampton. They sailed secretly at dusk, under the escort of destroyers, for Cherbourg, Brest, and as far south as Nantes and Saint-Nazaire in the Bay of Biscay.

Their speed of mobilization was impressive, as was the acceptance by everyone that nurses of all three services were ready, willing and able to share the hazards of active service. War was no longer a male monopoly.

British general hospitals, arriving in France, set up their wards, made modifications and changed locations according to instructions from headquarters British Expeditionary Force and with guidance from matron-in-chief, Miss Roy, at the War Office and principal matron, Miss Jones, in France. Moves were frequent. 'Once there were eight of us crammed into the back of an ambulance each time we moved. No one seemed to know what to do with us. Once we were on the move for three days,' said Lorna Kite who had landed at Dieppe.[2]

At last most hospitals in France settled into a routine. And then they waited. What were they to do now? The British soldier that autumn was physically fit; clement weather had kept them free from sickness. The fighting war had not yet begun. Nothing seriously disturbed the tenor of life in France or England. The terrifying air raids predicted, with thousands of casualties, had not materialized, and the Western Front had not yet developed. Only Poland had been attacked. It was the time of the Phoney War, as the press soon dubbed those months of inactivity after Poland had been defeated. Faced with the situation which Sister Joan Lister described as 'all dressed up and no-where to go', hospitals in France resorted to imaginative ways of keeping their medical staff occupied. One hospital in the Calvados region of Normandy made itself useful by opening an out-patients department for local French citizens. Nurses of another hospital took on the duties of a district nurse, visiting homes of those too ill to visit the hospital itself.

In Britain, then, hospitals were desperately trying to recruit more young women for training as nurses, for it was soon evident that many civilian nurses were being drawn away from civilian hospitals to the Navy, Army and Air Force nursing services. To fill their places recruits came from all walks of life. In the Great Ormond Street children's hospital, student nurse Selassie was in fact Princess Tsahia, daughter of the emperor of Abyssinia. Grateful patients in the London University College hospital would often turn to the tall, blue-eyed blonde who had dealt so efficiently with their injuries and ask if anyone had ever told her how like the Duchess of Kent she looked. 'You'd look just as pretty if you had the same lovely clothes,' said one man. And Nurse Kay, as she was called, just smiled. 'The secret of her identity was well kept. For she was, indeed, the Duchess of Kent, Princess Marina,' recalled Alec Adamson.[3]

Apart from trying to provide more nurses, hospitals also prepared for wartime demands by making more wards and beds available to cater for the thousands of domestic casualties expected hourly. At the Royal Herbert hospital at Woolwich, named after Sidney Herbert who had been so helpful to Florence Nightingale during the Crimean War, six more wards were quickly opened for the expected rush of wounded from air raids and battles in France.

Ready to receive those casualties at the reception office was Alec Adamson, a regular soldier in the RAMC. 'It was a huge hospital well staffed with QAIMNS nurses headed by a matron. We tended to be rather in awe of the QAs but I'm sure there was no need to be for they were always very pleasant and helpful. They were not the "battleaxes" that they were sometimes reputed to be.'

Dame Katherine Jones, matron-in-chief of the Army Nursing Service, would not have used the term 'battleaxes' to describe her nurses, but nevertheless she did not want them looked upon as 'ministering angels' either. It was part of her strategy for gaining commissioned-officer status for her fully qualified registered nurses that they be regarded firstly as soldiers and then as nurses. She believed that military nursing sisters should display an image more of masculine efficiency than of tender femininity if their true worth were to be recognized in the army. With this no doubt in mind she once said that if she were to be remembered in the history of nursing, she would be known as the 'militarizing Matron-in-Chief'.[4]

In 1941 she achieved her objective with full commissioned-officer status being granted to military registered nurses. Dame Katherine also recognized the invaluable contribution made to the whole nursing commitment by members of the Voluntary Aid Detachments.

Alec Adamson remembers them too: 'Those ladies in the VAD were hard working. One of them with us was Lady Anne Bowes, a cousin of the Queen Mother, who was, before her marriage to King George the Sixth, Lady Elizabeth Bowes Lyon.'

It is clear from Vera Brittain's book *Testament of Youth* that in the First World War there was a good deal of antagonism between the

QAs and the VADs, but I did not see any of this at all in the Royal
Herbert. Quite certainly, the hospital could not have functioned without the help of the VADs. No doubt, with their powerful aristocratic
links, many VAD nurses often tended to enjoy a kind of 'off-duty'
officer status.

Whatever the politics might have been about the blurring of
distinctions between registered and non-registered nurses, what
became quite clear was the invaluable contribution that wartime
VADs made to the general provision of nursing care. This increased
rapidly as the war went on, as Alec Adamson found.

At first, in that September of 1939, our patients came in dribs and
drabs. A crusty Captain Delgado kept us on our toes.

One night we had a soldier from the Pioneer Corps admitted
with appendicitis. He was on a stretcher, fully dressed with great-
coat, battle-dress, boots and gaiters. We laid him on the examination
couch and called out the duty medical officer. We peeled off all the
patient's clothing to reveal a well-fed, very hairy body. The medical
officer started to examine him and then suddenly backed off. The
soldier was crawling with crabs, the army term for pubic lice. We
had to shave and disinfect him from neck to the ankles.

For the first few months at the Royal Herbert all our patients
were similar to those coming in to any civilian hospital. Then in the
summer of 1940 things changed suddenly. Nurses found themselves
faced with a new set of instructions. They were written in German!

Sister Sheila McDermott (later Bambridge) remembers grappling
with the anglicized pronunciation of 'Haben Sie Schmerzen?' – 'Are
you in pain?'; 'Zeigen Sir Ihre Zunge' – 'Put out your tongue'; and 'der
Stuhlgang' – 'bowel movement' among a page full of other 'useful
expressions'. The reason for all this efficient preparation soon became
apparent as stretchers carrying German aircrew shot down over
London were brought in.

Sheila McDermott was put in charge of the Luftwaffe officers'
ward in the Royal Herbert, and she, along with her colleagues, soon
found that most German flyers were little different from their counterparts in the RAF. And just as the front-line soldiers on the Western
Front at Christmas 1914 treated each other like comrades in arms, so
too did nurses, staff and other patients of the hospital treat those
German aircrew.

But later in the war and immediately after it had ended, fraternization with prisoner-of-war patients became an offence for which

two sisters and one nurse were dismissed – sisters Margaret Mulvenna, aged 27, and Winnie Cunnane, 31, and Nurse Ivy Nott, from the Florence Nightingale Hospital, Bury. Then one 22-year-old German soldier, Werner Vetter was sentenced to twelve months' imprisonment for 'associating with a British girl'. This provoked such an outcry in the press and in parliament that War Minister Bellinger had to give in gracefully, saying, 'I have never attempted to resist the inevitable course of nature.' Vetter was reprieved, married Olive Reynolds at the village church 100 yards from the prisoner-of-war camp gates, accompanied by 150 guests and a German orchestra. Eight hundred marriages quickly followed.[5]

As Sheila Bambridge recalled, 'One could not help but become rather fond of some of them.' And the Germans did talk of the nurses as 'ministering angels attentive to our every need'. Yet every night German bombs were dropping around the hospital, filling its wards with mutilated bodies, horrifying nurses and medical orderlies alike.

> As a protection, all hospital windows were sprayed with a rubber solution but it did not prevent bits of glass from flying all over the place [recalled Alec Adamson]. One soldier was brought in having sustained a long jagged tear on his penis. We assisted the surgeon in inserting seventeen, yes seventeen, stitches in this vital part of the soldier's anatomy. No excitement for him until he had his stitches out![6]

During the deceptive lull on the Western Front that followed the German conquest of Poland, Britain and France had mounted a disastrous campaign in Norway. British nurses, dressed in man-sized winter clothing, cared for frost-bitten wounded soldiers above the Arctic Circle before being driven out of the country with the rest of the Norwegian Expeditionary Force. Nurses got back to Britain just before Hitler launched his 16,000 airborne troops and 136 divisions on 10 May 1940, to break through the Allied lines at lightning speed, hence the new word for the British public, 'Blitzkrieg'.

From the forward areas in France, over a thousand QA nurses under the control of principal matron Miss Jones, trekked back with BEF troops on roads dive-bombed and machine-gunned. 'I still have nightmares about those screeching German Stukas fitted with demonically blaring sirens which terrified us all,' recalled Sister Lorna Kite.[7]

In that hurried retreat, many hospitals had to destroy all their equipment prior to escape. Women of the FANY who had landed in

France with their senior commandant, Dr Joan Ince, in April 1940 drove night and day up to the very last moment ferrying wounded from casualty clearing stations to ports. Jagged holes in their ambulances testified to the times they had run the gauntlet along Luftwaffe-strafed roads. It was only when they heard the squeal of German tank tracks that they finally dashed at high speed for Saint-Malo, where they left their prized ambulances to be destroyed by a squad of sappers.

Caught in the confusion of operation orders was Miss F.M. Smith and nurses of 51st General Hospital, who had landed at Cherbourg on 20 May. She was sent south to Rennes and then told to join an ambulance train taking patients to a hospital ship at Saint-Nazaire. Soon after setting off, dive-bombers attacked the train and set fire to the carriage in which nursing sisters were travelling. The carriage was uncoupled and off they steamed again. They arrived at Saint-Nazaire in time to see the hospital ship sunk by dive-bombers – fortunately before patients were loaded. Miss Smith could hardly believe her eyes when she saw the same dive-bombers swoop down and machine-gun survivors in the water. She and her nursing colleagues sailed the next day in the *Duchess of York* and landed in Liverpool.[8]

Sister Elizabeth Williams of the hospital carrier *City of Paris* had been darting in and out of French ports for days. Particularly memorable for her was 2 June. As the ship was within sight of Dunkirk she went back to her cabin. Suddenly an almighty bang shook the ship and she was thrown across the cabin. Dazed, she recovered herself and felt her way to the door. There was shouting: 'Everyone on deck!' Once on the deck she heard a different instruction, 'All sisters in this boat'.

The engine room had been bombed. Once in the lifeboat she looked up and saw two German dive-bombers circling to attack. Then she was in the water as bombs exploded around her. She could hardly swim due to the weight of her clothes, and for thirty minutes she frantically struggled to keep afloat until she caught hold of a rope thrown over the side of the *City of Paris*. After experiencing great difficulty in hanging on to the rope she heard her commanding officer speak and was swiftly pulled into his lifeboat. More survivors were rescued in this way until at last a British tug took them all on board. 'The last to be taken out of our boat was a fourteen-year-old cabin boy curled up and apparently asleep. But he wasn't. He was dead,' wrote Sister Williams in her memoirs.

As soon as she had dried herself, she started to bandage the horrific burns received by men who had been in the engine room of the *City of Paris*. The tug was well on the way to Dover when German dive-bombers came again but then changed course. Sister Williams and her colleagues arrived in Dover six hours later where they boarded a hospital train. A short while later she joined Bolingbroke hospital.[9]

Sister Kite was with Number 5 Casualty Clearing Station, when they received orders to pack immediately and drive to Dunkirk.

Shells were already falling near us so we packed at speed, drove all day and at dusk pulled into an old chateau where stretchers with wounded from another Casualty Clearing Centre were lying outside. I was wondering where we could find a corner in which to sleep when I felt a hand tugging at my skirt. I looked down at the grey-faced lad lying on the stretcher by my feet. He looked vaguely familiar. Then I remembered. I knelt beside him. He had been a medical student in the hospital where I'd trained. He'd failed his medical exams and joined the Airforce. He was then a Sergeant Pilot and crashed near Fravent. He had a fractured femur and looked as though he'd lost a lot of blood. I was talking to him, making a note of his home address so that I could write to his parents, when the Matron interrupted me. Unbelievably she told me I was an officer and should not be chatting to a Sergeant – crass stupidity. His father was a Harley Street surgeon. It made me so angry. I later learnt that on his arrival at base they took off his plaster and his femoral artery bust. I often reproach myself for not taking a message from him to his parents. It's something I've lived with for a long time – poor John.[10]

Maybe that matron had been listening too closely to her matron-in-chief, Dame Katherine Jones, preaching the importance of QAIMNS nursing sisters safeguarding their status as officers assimilated into the army hierarchy.

But in June 1940 more important matters occupied the mind of nursing sisters withdrawing in haste to French evacuation ports. Many of the patients taken aboard had been prepared by the 'closed plaster' method, developed in the Spanish Civil War. All devitalized tissue around the wound was cut away, the wound left open and the cavity filled with a plain sterile vaseline pack. The whole limb would then be enclosed in a plaster cast including joints above and below, thus ensuring complete immobilization. The wound would not be inspected for ten days and some reports said thirty days was all right. Nurses found the limb developed an offensive odour and when the plaster was removed to cleanse the wound it was not unusual to find the job had already been done by a batch of fat maggots.

Incidentally, a report in the *Daily Telegraph* of 26 July 2000 told of a West Cumberland NHS Hospital placing 150 maggots on an open wound and leaving them to feed for three days. It was called larval therapy and reckoned to be the most effective form of treatment, as well as the cheapest. The closed plaster treatment in 1940 also made transportation of the wounded much easier and more comfortable for them.[11]

Whatever the method was in use it had to be done quickly in those last days of May 1940, for by the evening of the 23rd, German tank commanders could see the spires of Dunkirk. The way into the port was open. But those same commanders were astounded by orders to halt their advance. General Guderian protested – in vain. Hitler was adamant. The miracle of the Dunkirk evacuation began. Hitler had saved the BEF, the only trained army Britain possessed. Why? The decision has puzzled military historians ever since.

Some say Hitler was persuaded by Goering, who wanted his German Air Force to make the British surrender. 'My Führer, let my Luftwaffe deal with this. It will leave not one brick upon another. Not a man will escape the bombing of my Stukas! Our land forces will thus be spared unnecessary losses!'[12]

Off shore, and in northern French ports, ships were under constant attack. In Saint-Nazaire two hospital ships, *Maid of Kent* and *Brighton*, berthed alongside a tanker, went up in flames while patients were being taken on board. On the morning of 17 June 1940, Sister Lorna Kite was waving to thousands of troops packing the decks of HMT *Lancastria*, when it was hit by enemy bombs. It sank within four minutes. Only later was the death toll published – nearly 3,000 men drowned, equal to the combined losses of the *Lusitania* and the *Titanic* disasters. Churchill confessed later in his memoirs that he put a stop on all reporting of that loss and 'conveniently' forgot to take it off for fear of damaging public morale.

German pilots could see on the beaches between La Panne and Dunkirk hundreds of thousands of men, looking like black columns that wound their way from the sand dunes into the sea. There they stood chest-deep, waiting stoically for their turn to board small boats brought from moorings all over the south of England to take them on to destroyers off shore.

When some nurses reached Dunkirk it was already a flaming ruin. They made their way to the quays through smoke and heat, along streets strewn with the debris of houses that had collapsed. The corpses of dead horses, with gas-distended bellies, their legs sticking into the air, gave off a stench of putrefaction. One of the last of the QA nursing sisters to leave the beaches of Dunkirk was Lillian

Gutteridge (later Yarde-Martin). The men in her care were too severely wounded to wade out to the rescue boats and she was loading the stretches on to ambulances when German SS infantrymen captured her. The SS officer decided to take the ambulance and ordered his men to throw the wounded on to the ground. At this barbaric act Lillian became so angry she slapped the SS officer across the face. He drew his dagger and stabbed her in the thigh. Before he could plunge it anywhere else Sergeant McCracken with men from the Black Watch arrived and, to quote from Lillian's recent obituary in the QARANC Gazette, 'dispensed with the SS officer and helped reload the wounded into the ambulance'.[13]

Lillian drove to the railway siding, persuaded the French driver to take her wounded on board and they steamed away from Dunkirk towards Cherbourg, picking up over 600 British and French wounded along the way. Within a few days she and her wounded arrived safely back in England. This was one of the many miracles during that incredible evacuation.

Waiting for the severely wounded were 7,000 empty beds in hospitals close to the ports, and for those able to travel further there were beds in sector hospitals in Kent and Sussex. Mobile surgical teams with trained theatre nurses and student dressers were ready to be deployed to hospitals needing help.

In the seven days ending at midnight on 2 June 1940, there were 338,226 men evacuated from beaches at Dunkirk and La Panne by 222 Royal Naval ships and 665 civilian craft. Four years were to pass before nurses set foot in France again. Although the unexpected always happens in war, who in 1939 would have dared to say that France would withstand a German attack for barely a month? Now Britain was at bay, about to be invaded. German assault barges gathered in French ports.

On 15 September 1940, the German Luftwaffe launched a massive air attack against London and every major city, hoping to raze them all to the ground and break the people's will to carry on the war. Already some British politicians and the former King Edward, Duke of Windsor, wanted to make peace with Hitler. Edward, who had abdicated in order to marry Wallis Simpson, had well-known fascist sympathies and could easily have been amenable to overtures from Hitler.[14]

But Churchill and the British people were resolute. They would see the job through to the end, no matter how massive the air raids might be. Now every man, woman and child was a potential victim of sudden death from the skies.

Nurses played a valiant role during the next few months of the intensive air attacks, when over 500 hospitals were hit in raids on almost every city as well as in London. In the new Westminster hospital, while bombs were wrecking wards, operating theatres and all the latest equipment, nurses carried patients to safety and dowsed incendiary bombs with shovelfuls of sand and water from stirrup pumps. In Sheffield the whole staff helped to rescue patients during a heavy raid. In doing so the medical superintendent, his wife and the hospital matron were killed. Bombs fell directly on the nurses' home at Manchester Royal Infirmary, but fortunately all were then on the wards with their patients. At the neighbouring hospital, the Royal Hospital Salford, fourteen nurses were killed. A memorial to them was laid by the Duchess of Kent.

In Bristol, where bombs hit the Children's Hospital, nurses carried children in their arms and on their backs down to the shelters. 'Amazingly,' said one nurse, 'the children were marvellous! They were excited and singing in the shelter "Roll out the Barrel!" '

When bombs hit a hospital in Plymouth, nurses formed a chain, passing buckets of water up the stairs to a nurse who had clambered on to the roof rafters, dowsing incendiary bombs that had come through the slates. 'I'm not coming down until I've put out this fire!' the nurse shouted down to anxious colleagues calling for her.[15]

The blast from the bomb that hit the Royal Chest Hospital in London filled wards with dust so thick it was almost impossible to breathe or see where the patients were. However, Dr Bathfield, Matron McGovern and Staff Nurse Patricia Marmion immediately set about treating patients, pacifying them and moving wounded to wards where their injuries could receive better treatment. Patricia Marmion had to drag one patient away from a window from which he wanted to throw himself. Though bleeding profusely from a wound herself, she got him across her shoulders and carried him downstairs over masses of debris. She then went back to the ward to take the dangerous drugs to a safe place. Only then did she collapse and was taken to a bed in Grovelands Hospital. They had just got her to bed there when bombs hit that hospital. Windows were blown in and fires started. Nurse Marmion immediately began to help patients to safety, walking over shattered glass in her bare feet.

Two VAD nurses off duty in their Sussex village rescued the district nurse from her cottage and carried her to the village hall while bombs continued to fall. There the district nurse was killed outright by another bomb, and the two VAD nurses, Heather Barnes and Gertrude Pitceathly, were severely injured. Later they both were commended for their courage. 'Death is a mere incident in this struggle,' wrote the leader writer of the *British Journal of Nursing* then.

For fifty-seven nights continuously, from 7 September to 3 November 1940, the mightiest air assault ever raged over the fire-reddened skies of London. Wave after wave of bombers dropped thousands of tons of high explosive and incendiary bombs on the heart of the city. Nurses never had time to rest.

Neither did women ambulance drivers. Three of them were among the first women to receive the George Medal for outstanding bravery. They were Dorothy Clarke, Bessie Hepburn and Sonia Vera Carlyle, who drove their ambulances night after night through London streets while buildings tumbled and blazed.

It was not just nurses in hospitals who showed such courage. When the Luftwaffe attacked munition factories, staff nurses stayed at their posts. For example, Marjorie E. Perkins, a works nurse at Coventry, was flung across the works' surgery by the blast of the first bomb and though injured internally, she refused to seek safety in the air-raid shelter until she had attended to those lying bleeding on the factory floor. While tending them, another bomb knocked her unconscious, but she recovered and though in great pain carried on dealing with casualties. Her valour also earned her the George Medal.

The George Cross and George Medal decorations were created by King George VI in September 1940 especially for those displaying exceptional fortitude and outstanding gallantry during the air bombardment. In those critical times many civilians faced greater dangers than their compatriots in the armed forces. Indeed, up to September 1941 more civilians were killed than servicemen.

The first woman to win the George Cross was Daphne Pearson, a member of sick quarters staff at RAF Detling. Sleeping fitfully one night she heard an aircraft returning with its engine cutting out. She got up, dressed and ran out of her hut in time to see the plane crash nearby. She dashed to the aircraft, already on fire and dragged the pilot clear. Though injured he mumbled for her to get clear herself because there was a full load of bombs on board. She pulled him further away to the other side of a ridge just as the petrol tanks blew up. Daphne threw herself on top of the pilot to protect him from flying splinters and put her helmet over his head. As she lay over him a 120-pound bomb exploded. Other bombs exploded, but Daphne went back to the wreckage to look for the wireless operator. She found him dead.

At eight o'clock the next morning she was on duty as usual. Daphne died in July 2000, aged eighty-nine.

That was the spirit of those days. People refused to be cowed. They would not give in. The more intensive the bombing, the greater their resolution grew. Nowhere was this spirit exemplified more than on the horrific night of terror when Hitler attempted to raze Coventry to the ground.

It had been a mild cloudless day, and the night was star-studded and lit by a full moon. It was Friday, 14 November 1941. The warbling notes of the air-raid siren sounded, then the yellow warning light flashed on the wards of Coventry and Warwickshire hospital. Nurses knew it meant: 'Danger imminent, go to action stations.'

Through the windows nurses could see why. The whole sky was alight from pathfinder chandelier flares dropped by throbbing German bombers looking for their munition works targets. Every building was bathed in a pure white incandescent glow. Bombs came whistling down. Incendiaries followed the high explosives.

Matron Joyce Burton responded immediately in her usual brisk manner. Immaculate as a Guards sergeant-major, her tightly fitting purple dress wrinkle-free, her starched white collar precisely centred above the middle pleat of her dress, she walked swiftly to the nearest of her wards – emergency or not, matrons do not run – to see for herself that the action stations drills were carried out. Joyce Burton left nothing to chance.

In the medical ward Sister Emma Horne, a dark-haired Welsh woman, pushed her glasses up the bridge of her nose and uttered her strongest expletive: 'Well, drat my buttons!'

Neither of these two women looked like the type seen in films, who would throw caution to the winds and perform heroic deeds. Yet in the real-life drama of that long, horrific night, both of them earned one of the highest civilian awards for valour: the George Medal.

Within minutes, hundreds of incendiary bombs spluttered round the hospital, their white flames setting ablaze anything combustible. Fires started in many parts of the hospital. Sister Betti Price (now Howe) was in the bath in the nurses' home when the first incendiary fell. 'I had to grope about in the dark to find some clothes to put on.'[16] The nurses' home was soon blazing.

By that time Betti was attempting to pacify patients in her ophthalmic ward. 'They were mainly elderly men and women who usually had to lie quite still after their operations, but we managed to put them into wheel chairs and get them down to the ground floor. There were put them on beds with a mattress on top of them as some sort of cover from flying glass and masonry.'

In the courtyard, doctors and nurses ignored the whizzing shrapnel

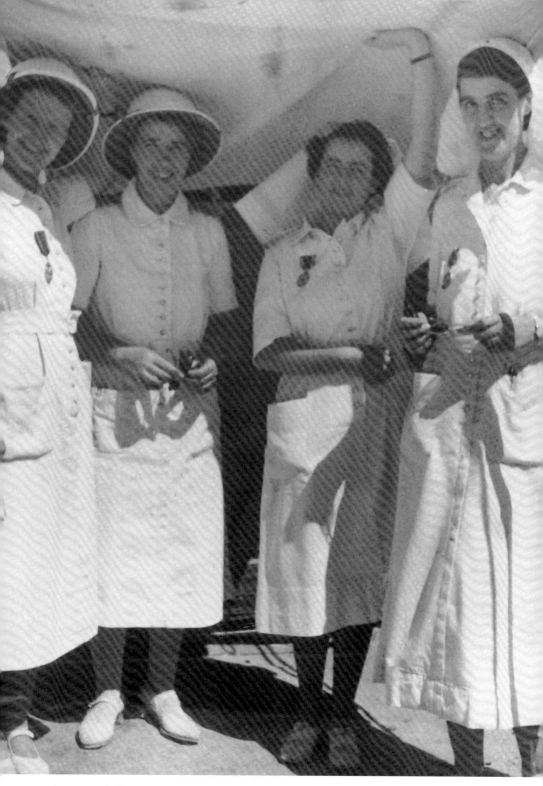

Matron and three nursing sisters of QAIMNS serving in the Middle East
(photograph courtesy of the Imperial War Museum, London)

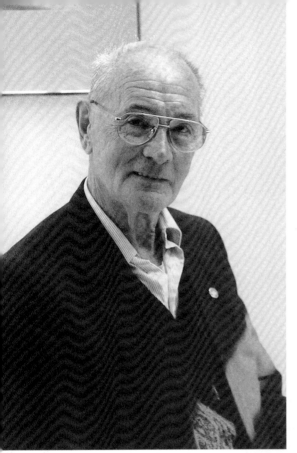

Derek Ball, a casualty at Anzio, described the nurses at the casualty clearing station on the beachhead as 'marvellous, calm and reassuringly wonderful'

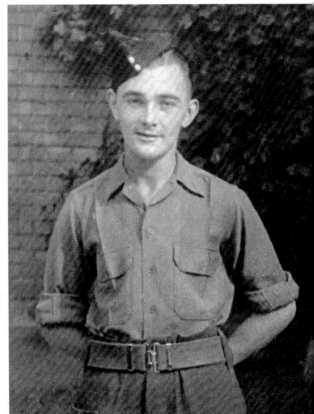

Derek Ball in battledress and side cap, 1944

Freda Barnfather QAIMNS (now Reid) served in the Sudan and on hospital ships. Excessive exposure to the sun meant that skin surgery was necessary in later life

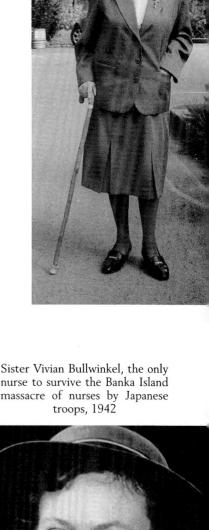

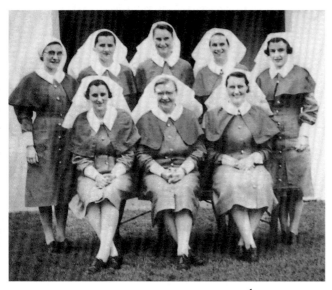

Some victims of the Japanese Army: 2/4th Casualty Clearing Station, 1942. Front row (*from left*) Staff Nurse D. Gardam (POW, died 1945); Matron I. Drummond (shot Banka Island, 1942), Sister E.M. Hannah (POW); back row (*from left*) Staff Nurse E. Dorsch (drowned 1942); Staff Nurse B. Willmott (shot Banka Island, 1942); Staff Nurse W. Raymont (POW died 1945); Sister Balfour-Ogilvy (shot Banka Island, 1942); and Staff Nurse P. Farmaner (shot Banka Island, 1942)

Sister Vivian Bullwinkel, the only nurse to survive the Banka Island massacre of nurses by Japanese troops, 1942

Sister Beatrice Hownam survived the sinking of the troopship 'Strathallen' in which five nurses lost their lives

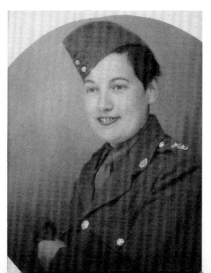

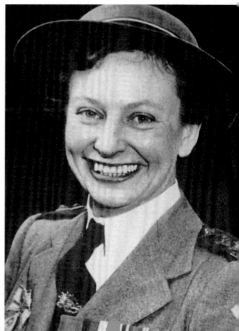

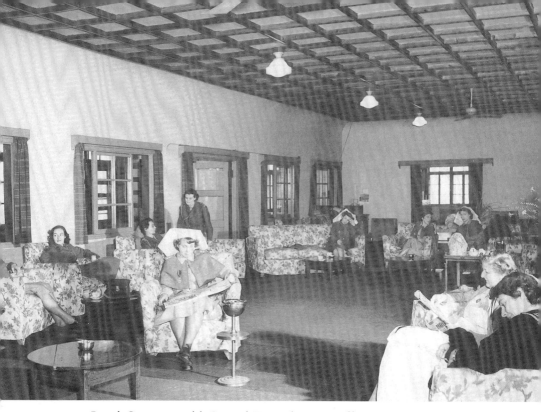

British Commonwealth General Hospital, women officers' mess ante room, Kure, Japan. (Sister Jill McNair *centre*)

QARANC cloak belonging to Jill McNair, with its collection of military badges mainly from patients. This was rather frowned upon by the powers that be. However, many years later the same cloak was on display at the National Army Museum's Korean exhibition. 'I still have the cloak – now fifty years old', says Jill

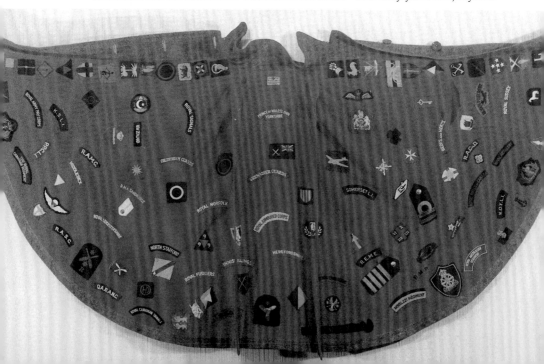

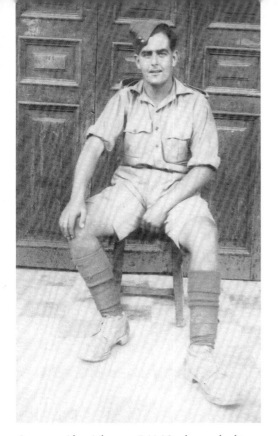

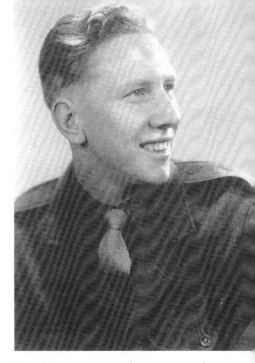

David Oates, a national serviceman who served in Britcom General Hospital, Kure, Japan, during the Korean War as a member of the operating team

Sergeant Alec Adamson RAMC who worked in military hospitals in Britain and the Middle East throughout the war said, 'I saw the brutality of war at first hand. I came back safely but the reality of the words "they died that we might live" still comes home to me. Merely to thank them for their sacrifices seems inadequate. We must take positive action to prevent it ever happening again. As I have got older my memories of those whom I saw die are of young men and women, and the words "they will never grow old" have become more poignant and meaningful. Yes, *we* will always remember them'

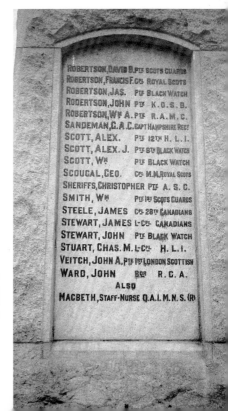

War memorials throughout Britain carry names of nurses who lost their lives in the South African wars and both world wars, as this one in Pitlochry does

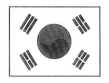

## 존경하는

6·25전쟁이 발발한지 반세기를 맞아 세계의 자유 민주주의와 대한민국을 수호하는데 기여한 귀하에게 진심으로 감사드립니다. 아울러 고귀한 생명을 바치신 영령앞에 무한한 경의와 추모의 뜻을 표합니다.

대한민국이 오늘날의 자유 민주주의 국가를 유지할 수 있도록 귀하께서 보여주셨던 불굴의 신념과 진정한 용기, 그리고 거룩한 희생정신을 우리는 가슴속 깊이 간직하고 있습니다.

특히 귀하께서 50년전에 몸으로 실천했던 자유민주주의 이념은 이제 새로운 세기, 새 천년을 맞아 세계 인류의 보편적 가치가 되었습니다.

이에 6·25전쟁 50주년을 맞이하여 귀하의 명예를 드높임과 동시에 과거 혈맹으로 맺어졌던 귀하와의 우의를 재다짐하고자 합니다. 아울러 인류의 발전과 평화를 위해 세계 우방들과 함께 노력해 나갈 것입니다.

다시 한번 귀하의 숭고한 헌신에 깊이 감사드리며 행운과 건승을 기원합니다.

감사합니다.

2000년 6월 25일

대 한 민 국 대 통 령       김 대 중

Letter of appreciation from the President o

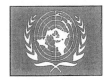

June 25, 2000

Dear Mu JuMclait,

On the occasion of the 50th anniversary of the outbreak of the Korean War, I would like to offer you my deepest gratitude for your noble contribution to the efforts to safeguard the Republic of Korea and uphold liberal democracy around the world. At the same time, I remember with endless respect and affection those who sacrificed their lives for that cause.

We Koreans hold dear in our hearts the conviction, courage and spirit of sacrifice shown to us by such selfless friends as you, who enabled us to remain a free democratic nation.

The ideals of democracy, for which you were willing to sacrifice your all 50 years ago, have become universal values in this new century and millennium.

Half a century after the Korean War, we honor you and reaffirm our friendship, which helped to forge the blood alliance between our two countries. And we resolve once again to work with all friendly nations for the good of humankind and peace in the world.

I thank you once again for your noble sacrifice, and pray for your health and happiness.

Sincerely yours,

Kim Dae-jung
President of the Republic of Korea

blic of Korea, Kim Dae-jung, 25 June 2000

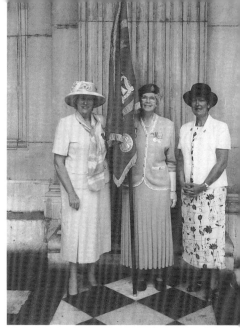

Mrs Jill McNair carrying the QARANC standard, with Lt.-Col. Margaret Nesbit RRC (Retd) and Major Diana Wilson (Retd), after the Korean Veterans Association International Reunion Service at St Paul's Cathedral, 19 July 1999

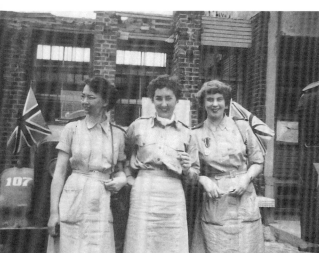

Three nursing sisters, QARANC, outside Britcom Z Hospital, Seoul, Korea, on Coronation Day, 2 June 1953. (Sister Jill Hall, now McNair, *on right*)

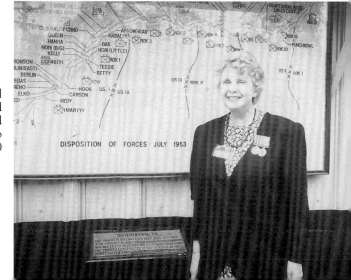

Return to Korea. Jill McNair outside the United Nations Command Advance HQ, Camp Boniface, September 1990

from the anti-aircraft shells and the incendiaries dropping around them, as they ferried patients from the outside temporary wards to the main building. Sister Gladys Crichton was at the end of a stretcher, carrying a man with leg injuries. Partly to fortify herself, as well as her patient, she said to him: 'It won't be long now, Dad.' He replied, 'Less of the Dad. I'm not even married.' She has always remembered how jolly he was, lying on the stretcher looking up into the sky saying, 'Hey, look at the fairy lights!'

One patient, Mrs Evans of Green Lane, Coventry, then recovering from a major operation, could not find enough words of praise for those nurses.

They pulled beds away from the windows, put wash-basins over our heads to protect us from flying debris and when an incendiary bomb fell through the window one of them ran to put it out with sand and got burnt in the process. And then when a bomb blew part of the wall away the nurses pushed the beds into a long corridor between the wards. Then there was another very loud explosion and part of the ceiling came down on us. The bombing went on until daybreak. At last came the quiet. The longed for wail of the 'All Clear' siren. Peace.[17]

In that one night of terror, all the city's essential services were put out of action, fire hydrants buried under piles of masonry, water mains shattered by bombs, and the mains gas and electricity supplies cut off, causing additional problems in the hospital. As Sister Gladys Crichton recalled:

In Casualty we worked with paraffin lamps – ironically stamped 'Made in Germany' – and used Dettol to keep needles, sutures and swabs sterile. Our first casualties were firemen who had approached incendiary bombs just as they burst hurling fragments of hot metal which embedded themselves in their faces and hands. We just had to probe bits out and stitch them up. Then many of them went back on duty again.

Some casualties were so mutilated they were beyond any treatment and they were just given injections of pain killing morphia. The dead were lying amongst the dying and the living. And those who were waiting could see what was happening. Many of the wounded on stretchers looked no different from the dead. In fact this caused a problem with one elderly lady who had an open wound on her scalp that I could not cope with adequately in Casualty. I was taking her to the Out Patients Department where there were better facilities. As we entered the room she took one look and shouted, 'I'm not going in there, they're all dead.' The only way I could convince her they were alive was to ask all those lying on stretchers to raise their arms and show the lady she was indeed amongst the living. Only then did she consent to being taken in. I shaved her head, incised the black edges of her wound and stitched it together.

Surgeon Harry Winter worked all through the night using emergency lighting when the mains electricity failed and then by the light of a car's headlamp when the emergency generator ceased to function. He recalled, 'Every few minutes the nurses and anaesthetist threw themselves under the operating table as bombs roared down close to the hospital.'

Throughout that night, Matron Joyce Burton never once sat down. She walked the wards reassuring younger nurses, inspiring them, questioning in a quiet manner, listening and making positive suggestions. By morning she was no longer immaculate. Her face, at any other time, would have been thought a ludicrous sight – smutty, smoke-stained, begrimed; a grotesque mask. But it exuded confidence and a feeling that everything was under control. And the nurses responded well to the challenge.

How did those young women, many just out of their teens, manage to do it? Sister Betti Price, reflecting on that night recalled her own strange reaction.

It was frightening yet in a way I felt detached from it, like an onlooker at some frightful drama. I remember one time in the middle of the raid, snatching a quick cup of tea and I saw a curtain catch fire and swing lazily in the night breeze blowing in through the shattered windows. And the funny thing was I took it as nothing exceptional or frightening. Perhaps it was because I was young or just numbed. It was my twentieth birthday.

Surgeon Harry Winter was amazed by the way nurses carried on calmly. 'The morale of everyone was stupendous. The emergency galvanized the whole hospital. Bombs thundered down but after a time few nurses even bothered to duck! There was not one cry of fear. Not one case of hysteria all night.'

As Probationer Nurse Edna Vine walked through the city of Coventry on her way to the hospital the next morning she could hardly believe her eyes. Fires burned all over the ruined city. There was no water. Even the canal, breached by bombs, had been drained. The raid gave a new verb to the German language: *koventrieren* – to coventrate, that is, to annihilate or raze to the ground. That night, twenty-seven vital war factories were hit, a firestorm started and burnt out more than a square mile of the city centre, 60,000 of the 75,000 buildings were destroyed and 568 men, women and children killed.

In the Coventry and Warwickshire hospital, most of the windows were gone, walls had great gaps and hardly a door remained on its frame. The nurses' home was in ruins. But all was not yet over for nurses in that hospital. On 8 April another massive raid reduced the building to a mere shell, and this time nurses were left mourning their colleagues buried under heaps of bricks and charred timber. Some had been rescued and lay in the hospital as Betti Price remembers still: 'The girl who relieved me on night duty was dying. I was angry, blazing angry that she should be so young and dying. I spoke to the surgeon, wanting something to be done. He just looked at me for a moment, without speaking, and then said simply that nothing could be done. She was indeed, just dying.'

There was nothing to be done for the hospital then either. The building was wrecked, unusable. Matron Burton gave instructions to the nurses: 'If you have anywhere to go, leave your name and address and go. Just go.'

They could not all be given medals and so George Medals were given to their representatives – Matron Joyce Burton, Sister Emma Horne and the hospital house governor in recognition of everyone's extraordinary and gallant devotion to duty.

And of such mettle were nurses from all those 500 hospitals hit by bombs in 1940 and 1941. They had proved themselves and they would be just as resolute in facing the further challenges in 1944 when the flying bombs and V2 rockets rained down upon southern England.

Meanwhile another crisis had arisen. There was an acute shortage of nurses. In June 1940 Mussolini had declared war on Britain and France. Now British troops, with nurses in support, had been sent to the Middle East, where two of Italy's best armies were threatening Cairo and the Suez Canal.

# 14 Middle East Adventure

'Where do we go from here
Now that we've got Bardia?'
Popular song in Britain after a British victory
in the Western Desert of Libya

The New Year of 1941 found British troops fighting on three war fronts: in Libya, Greece and Eritrea. To each of them went nurses with their supporting field and general hospitals.

The first of these attacks was against the Italian stronghold of Bardia on the Libyan frontier. British and Australian soldiers attacked under the cover of a massive bombardment from the battleship *Valiant*. On board was a 19-year-old midshipman, Prince Philip of Greece, who would later become Duke of Edinburgh. The whole operation was short and highly successful. Bardia was taken and with it 35,000 Italian prisoners. And this gave British newspapers, music writers and the public something to sing about with the catchy song of 'Where do we go from here?'

Nurses in the Navy, Army, and Air Force were also wondering where they were going to go, for so many were being sent on embarkation leave. Matrons in civilian hospitals were also wondering where to go from here to find enough nurses for their own wards. So critical was the shortage of trained and experienced nurses in August 1940 that Lord Davies in the House of Lords called for conscription to direct women into training for nursing. And VIP guests at grammar school speech days were appealing to girls to take up nursing as a career. 'Go then. Choose your training school. Commence and persevere in your training,' said one speaker closing her address in Churchillian style in December 1941.[1]

Nurses in significantly increasing numbers now began to join the staffs of British military hospitals and hospital ships in the Middle East as the campaign against Italy gained momentum. On 22 January

1941 British and Australian troops surrounded Tobruk taking prisoner 25,000 Italian troops.

These were encouraging days for Britain. But not for long. Hitler, not wishing to see his Axis partner being defeated, sent his 15th Armoured Division to North Africa under one of his favourite generals, Rommel. Soon the port was under attack. Nurses were quickly moved into Tobruk to look after the wounded. Angela Rigby was with them:

> Some of us stayed with the hospital there. The town was in ruins including most of the hospital building. German bombers, newly based on Sicilian airfields, raided the town almost daily. Yet no one seemed to take much notice of the raids. There were no warnings. We had ten operating theatres going and stretcher bearers brought casualties into a large reception room and laid them side by side. Three or four medical officers moved up and down the lines picking out those needing immediate surgery. The next morning all casualties fit enough to travel were loaded onto a hospital ship or the ambulance convoy.
>
> The usual practice in the operating theatres was for one Sister to be scrubbed up with two instrument trolleys standing between two operating tables and for the Sister to assist whenever needed. We had no penicillin in those early days and nursing care was somehow more important.
>
> How I longed for the days when we had boiling water immediately available for sterilization instead of having to wait ages for a primus stove to boil the water in the drums. Some wounds were just so terrible there was little we could do for those poor lads but give them enough morphine to take away the pain. We gave equal care to the Germans as we did to our own. The front line was so fluid that sometimes we took into our care German wounded who had already been treated by their own doctors and we noted how often that treatment had meant a quick amputation. I suppose German surgeons were so busy at times they decided it took far longer to remove shrapnel and deal with fractures than to amputate a limb.[2]

Major Watts in his casualty clearing station had the same problem with wounded German soldiers who had first been treated by their own doctors. Many of them had had a 'guillotine amputation' which British surgeons considered as being totally unjustifiable because once the skin had healed the patient was left with an exposed bone. Furthermore, infection frequently set in and there was a good deal of subsequent pain. They regarded this 'guillotine' method as barbarous.[3]

Angel Rigby remembered cases of bone protruding through wounds she treated. In one instance a German gunner had sustained numerous shell fragment injuries. Three or four inches of the tibia was visible. The tissue around it had gangrene and it was crawling with maggots. In the Middle East flies could not be kept off wounds but both doctors and nurses found that maggots actually cleared away the decayed flesh. Flies were an annoyance for everyone. Whenever a meal was eaten, 'one hand had to be wafting them off the spoon as we lifted it to our lips,' wrote Angela.[4]

To Tobruk also at that time came a small company of women ambulance drivers of Number 11 Company of the Women's Transport Service, part of the First Aid Nursing Yeomanry. The ambulances were K2 Austins and the driver was protected from sun, wind and rain only by canvas screens. Fortunately for nurses and patients these ambulances had large tyres and heavy springs which enabled them to travel smoothly even over very rough ground. Each ambulance could take five stretcher cases.[5]

Evacuation of wounded was sometimes by sea to Malta but the island suffered terribly throughout the campaigns in the Western Desert and in Tunisia. Several naval and army hospitals were hit by bombs, some completely destroyed, with nurses and doctors killed in the intensive German air raids. So heavy was the bombing that Churchill 'fearing it would be pounded to bits' asked the United States to send the aircraft carrier *Wasp* to try again to deliver fighter aircraft to defend the island. The story of the courage shown by men and women during those months, for which they were awarded the George Cross in September 1942, is told more fully in my *Front-line Nurse*. But it was not all blood and guts for the nurses there. Somehow they managed to find time for amusement wherever they were.

British, Australian and New Zealand nurses were also being subjected to air bombardment in Greece, which had been invaded by Italian troops in October 1940, and joined later by fifteen German divisions. In response to a Greek appeal for help the Eighth Army dispatched a token force of 53,000 men, but neither they  nor the Greeks could hold the German onslaught. Within a short time they and their hospitals were hustled back to their evacuation ports and beaches in the south.

A British nurse graphically recounted the ordeal of those last few hours after they had driven without lights from Athens, at night, down roads cratered by bombing or shellfire, towards a small fishing harbour, and one bus had overturned. The nurses scrambled out of the wreckage and were packed into other buses. They drive by night and, by day, hid wherever they could in ruined buildings to dodge the dive-bombers. One day, when they were consuming their minuscule rations in a graveyard, they were detected by German aircraft that began attacking any moving object.

Eventually, as they neared the small harbour it was too dangerous to travel by bus, so in small groups they walked the last two miles dragging with them what little luggage they still had. One nurse fell into the water whilst boarding a Greek ship. Two sailors jumped in and wedged their backs against the walls and their feet against the ship to keep it away from them whilst ropes were dropped and all three were pulled clear and the ship sailed for Egypt.[6]

It was another Dunkirk! This time called 'Operation Demon'. In six days 50,732 men were evacuated from eight small ports. Nurses from the hospital at Larissa left all their equipment and baggage behind as they raced for the coast in front of German motorized troops. Nurses of No. 26 British General Hospital at Kifisia handed over their patients to Greek nurses and doctors and headed at full speed for the beach at Argos. There a Greek fishing boat took them off shore to an Australian destroyer. It was the same scenario all over southern Greece, where troops and nurses were being picked up under fire from German dive-bombers.

Most of the nurses were taken to Crete, where soon they had to go through the same evacuation experience again, as German airborne troops captured the island. Other nurses from Greece were taken directly to Alexandria.

There in the meantime, nurses arriving from Britain were taking the long journey south to hospitals in the Sudan. A large Italian army had occupied Kassala, a town inside Anglo-Egyptian Sudan. A force of 30,000 British and Sudanese troops had attacked the Italians in January 1941 and for five months had battled through rocky hills and thorn scrubland that favoured the defenders. Casualties were taken to military hospitals at Asmara and Gebeit, where more nurses were urgently needed. With them was Sister Monty Winstanley, who had just arrived after enjoying a wonderful tour of the Holy Land whilst on leave from the 54th General Hospital at Ismailia.

She and her colleagues had travelled two days down the Nile by river steamer, akin to an American showboat, for two days and nights. Then they boarded a train that stopped at sundown every evening to let the Muslims get off to pray facing Mecca. At this time locals would appear from nowhere selling hard-boiled eggs and fruit. The final part of the journey, as Monty described it, was by ten-ton truck, winding its way up the hills to Number 16 Combined General Hospital, Asmara, 8,000 feet above sea level. It was staffed by six QA sisters, a matron and Indian nursing sisters. Monty recalled that the worst things she had to contend with were rats and locusts, which flew at night and banged into the faces of anyone in their way. The best thing was, without doubt, the young officer whom she met there and married in September 1943.

In the Sudan also was medical technician Alec Adamson. He remembered clearly what it was like for nurses and staff stationed at the 59th General Hospital, Gebeit. Alec found it difficult to get accustomed to the arid heat and the occasional violent thunderstorms that turned the hospital and quarters into an island with raging torrents all around. The land dried quickly and the sandstorms would return. It was a relief to everyone when their turn came to use the small swimming pool near the camp. It had been excavated by Italian prisoners of war and had a drain plug fitted so that the water could be changed. As Alec Adamson remembered, it was refilled by a hundred prisoners, each carrying a five gallon can of water on his head trudging across the sand to the swimming pool.

I remember thinking at the time what a topsy turvy world we were living in where the mere whim of those in charge was satisfied by using the labour of hundreds of others. I learnt Italian and got quite fluent. There was a cinema at Gebeit about five miles away and we went there now and again.

Several of the lads had unusual pets, chameleons. They were kept on a piece of tree branch and restrained from wandering off by tying one end of a piece of string to the branch and the other to the hind leg of the animal. They were usually placed where there was a plentiful supply of flies and helped to keep the fly population of our tents down to a tolerable level.

The food for us was reasonably good but no fresh vegetables or meat. Corned beef, tinned bacon and porridge were plentiful but the bread was an acquired taste, for we had to get used to eating thousands of tiny weevils which infested the flour. We got used to the extra but unwanted protein.

The Sudanese locals were very honest and helpful. They would bring us things from the town, leave them with us until pay day and then collect the money. They did all our laundry, kept the tents tidy, cleaned our boots and made the beds. They were good tailors too and kept our shirts immaculately ironed. They took a swig of water, pursed their lips and sprayed surfaces to be moistened. Not very hygienic but effective nevertheless.[7]

The Italian armies in Eritrea were finally defeated with the surrender of Massawa and it was time for nurses in Sudan hospitals to be employed elsewhere. Some went to Iraq and some to Persia. It was little known then that some years before the war, Hitler dreamed and prepared for his *drang nach ost* (drive to the east) sending German engineers to improve and build new Persian railways. He infiltrated German engineers and scientists into Iraq also, at the same time encouraging Raschid Ali (an anti-British general who had seized power in Iraq on 2 April 1941) to plan a revolt against the British when the time was ripe. Hitler wanted the oil in the Persian Gulf now denied to him by Allied armies. In his quest for oil he also launched his armies against Stalingrad and the Caucasus, hoping to drive on to India.

In 1941, before the battles of Stalingrad had started, Hitler's plans were set back by the military cost of the Greek campaign and the defeat of the Vichy French in Syria – where British nurses had served also. Unfortunately for Hitler, his conspiring protégé in Iraq, Raschid Ali, started his revolt before German troops could give him support. Two British brigades put down his revolt and captured Baghdad. The revolt forced Allied high command to build up their Tenth Army in Basra to forestall further German attempts to advance there.

It was not long before British and Commonwealth nurses were sailing up the Persian Gulf to Basra. On board ships their white dresses were soaked with perspiration minutes after donning them. Yvonne Jeffrey, with colleagues from Number 1 General Hospital, Kantara, also travelled to Number 35 Combined British and Indian Hospital in the desert outside Tehran. They looked after Polish soldiers captured by the Russians after their occupation of part of Poland, in accordance with the Nazi–Soviet non-aggression pact of 23 August 1939. The prisoners were later released after Germany invaded Russia without warning on 22 June 1941. Incidentally, on that same day 129 years earlier Napoleon had invaded Russia hoping also for victory celebrations in Moscow.

It was a strange task for British nurses building those emaciated former prisoners up to strength. They responded well and were soon on their way to join Allied troops in Egypt.

In this limited space it is not possible to give detailed accounts of all these campaigns, but a few personal recollections can profitably merge into the common record. Gradually we can piece together a composite picture of what it was really like for those nurses in so many different campaigns. Their activities have already been chronicled in greater detail in the two previous books on wartime nurses by this writer.[8]

During the autumn of 1941 and spring 1942 the Eighth Army advanced and withdrew so often in the Western Desert that armchair tacticians could hardly keep their maps up to date. By November 1941 it had reached Tobruk but on 21 June 1942, 30,000 Eighth Army men surrendered to Rommel at Tobruk, leaving him with 2,000 vehicles in working order and 2,000 tons of petrol.

Alarmingly, by 1 July both German Panzer divisions were on the Egyptian frontier barely a morning's drive from Cairo. Sister Majorie Bennett, then nursing in Cairo, recalls meeting a crowd marching down the street chanting in a mixture of Arabic and English: 'We want Rommel. English go now!' Egyptians, confident of a German victory, tore down British flags and put up Nazi ones.

The city was in crisis. Hospitals were full. Women in all three services were told to be packed ready to embark at a moment's notice. Nurses were to stay with their patients in hospitals. Their presence was too good for morale for them to leave.

The two desert armies now faced each other at a point on the map marked with a small railway station called El Alamein. It was at this time that some nurses were undergoing a most unusual experience. They were on board the famous 30,000-ton *Queen Mary*, the world's largest liner. Launched in 1934, the ship made headline news before the war by earning the 'Blue Riband' for the fastest crossing of the North Atlantic. Now it was playing a vital role in saving the desperate position at El Alamein. She was sailing at full speed from the United Kingdom to Port Suez, crammed with troops that were quartered in every conceivable part of the ship, and with nurses and American tanks, for the depleted Eighth Army. Too fast for the U-boats, at one time speeding through a pack of twenty-five of them, it covered the 12,000-mile voyage round the Cape in record time. Its complement of men and nurses arrived in good time to take up their positions for the first battle of El Alamein on 1 July 1942, which halted Rommel's armies.

More nurses moved forward during August and September and were ready to receive casualties from the even more decisive battle that followed. It began on a bright moonlit night on 23 October with a shattering bombardment from 900 guns, firing with maximum intensity for fifteen minutes. Then the infantry advanced through the minefields onto German machine-guns. And the nurses knew what that must have been like. Sister Margaret Jennings remembers the shock of receiving those casualties:

> Stretcher followed stretcher of wounded, bewildered and blood-caked soldiers: some who'd been half-roasted alive in tanks, heads and faces blasted by shells and bullets. Many with limbs missing too. And so many bleeding still who'd already had blood transfusions from the mobile unit nearer the front. The urgency of the tasks lent skill to our fingers. Bandages, sticky with blood and sand were removed, bleeding stopped, and wounds redressed. Infected wounds were treated and Plaster of Paris applied where advised by medical officers.
>
> The expressions of relief and gratitude on their faces when they sank incredulously onto beds was unforgettable. The courage and fortitude of those lads was such an example and inspiration to us all. Somehow though, despite the shock of the experience, the feelings of horror, compassion and awe were mixed with something akin to a glow of satisfaction that we had been able to do something really worthwhile for them. We were doing what, all that time ago, we had set out to do. And though we did not admit it at the time, there was a great feeling of humility mixed with pride in all this.[9]

When the five-day battle was over, the German and Italian forces were in swift retreat. They had lost 2,300 men killed and 27,900 taken prisoner. General Montgomery was suddenly famous. 'It is a strange experience,' he wrote in his *Memoirs*, 'to find oneself famous and it would be ridiculous to deny that it was rather fun.' The price of Montgomery's 'fun' was 13,500 killed, missing and wounded from the Eighth Army. Nurses who went forward with the Eighty Army received a special letter of appreciation from the matron-in-chief, Middle East, Dame Katherine Jones: 'We know how your have advanced with the victorious troops and also how you have worked at high pressure in base hospitals. We know also how difficult it is for you nursing men of different creeds and languages.'

West of Alamein, British and Commonwealth forces continued to drive the Germans and Italians from their North African conquests. And then to Hitler's dismay came news of an Allied force landing in Iran and Algiers – the largest amphibious invasion force known in the history of warfare – and it was attacking German troops hurriedly dispatched to defend Tunis.

It was while the fighting in Tunisia was at its bloodiest, with armies battling for possession of Longstop Hill and with casualties overflowing the corridors of the 98th British General Hospital, Algiers, that a most oddly dressed man in his early sixties walked into the surgical ward. He wore a panama hat and long khaki shorts that covered his white knees. The stranger was Professor Alexander Fleming. He had arrived to supervise personally the administering of his new drug, penicillin.

Though the drug was discovered by the British bacteriologist in 1929, it had not before been used for septic wounds. Commercial production of this new 'wonder drug' was developed by Ernest Chain and Howard Florey. All three men would share the Nobel Prize in 1945 in recognition of their work.

In that April, of 1943, doctors and nurses marvelled at the drug's effect on soldiers with repulsive wounds infected with gas gangrene. Almost incredibly, these patients began to recover. The new yellow powder, smelling of 'old hay', began to revolutionize the treatment of wounds. Nurses working with this new drug during the next few weeks, as casualties continued to pour into hospitals, had the satisfaction of seeing for themselves the tremendous effect it had on the death and disability rate. It was a real boost to everyone's morale in overcrowded, overworked hospitals.

Thousands of soldiers were spared the life-threatening amputations occasioned by gas gangrene and other infections. And although supplies were limited it was nevertheless used with patients suffering from venereal diseases, on the grounds that these men could be cured quickly by the drug and returned to their fighting units, where they were desperately needed in the latter years of the war.

It was also used to cure Prime Minister Winston Churchill when he fell ill with pneumonia on his visit to North Africa. His recovery was further testimony to the wonders of penicillin. 'The great change to nursing came with this new drug,' recalled Marie Floyd Norris. 'Such was its effect that we even began to think that our good nursing care might not have as much to do with recovery as it used to do.'[10]

Nurses could not help speculating whether or not it was the availability of the drug that led to a surprising decision by the government then. From the autumn of 1943, the recruitment of experienced nurses from the civilian sector to the military nursing services was officially restricted. Only newly qualified nurses could join up. The decision could also have been made because civilian hospitals were beginning to lack well-qualified and experienced registered nurses.

In Africa, though, there was still plenty to keep them busy. Some patients, such as those with severe facial wounds, required almost constant attention, as Alec Adamson recalled:

We had three patients all at one time suffering serious injuries to the throat needing the insertion of a tracheotomy tube just below the thyroid cartilage of the Adam's Apple. There were actually two tubes. The first tube was inserted into the trachea so that the flanged edge rested on the surface of the next and was kept in place by two pieces of tape passing round the neck. In this way the tube was not ejected if the patient coughed. Into the outer tube was placed a smaller flexible tube which allowed air to enter the lungs without going through the mouth and nose. This inner tube had to be removed and cleaned at frequent intervals. Feeding was a problem too because the patient could not take solid food. Liquid feeding was done by using a Ryle's tube passed into the stomach. All this took a great deal of time and other patients had to have less.

Two of the patients recovered satisfactorily but the third case, a Guardsman, had been badly wounded in the Mareth Line battle. His right arm was missing and most of the front of his neck had been shot away. His tracheotomy tube and feeding tube were in place but although he was unable to speak we tried to understand what he was attempting to convey to us. In spite of his critical condition he kept smiling, trying to be cheerful even. He began to have difficulty in breathing and fluid was gathering in his right lung. The surgeon took out a section of rib and inserted a drainage tube. His condition worsened and one afternoon when we had drawn the blinds to keep the room cool, he signalled that he wanted the blinds taken away. He smiled and nodded his thanks when I did it and I sensed he was dying and asking for more light. I have often thought that I should get in touch with his parents and tell them how brave their son was. Every armistice day I think of Guardsman J—— of the Grenadiers and the sacrifice he and others made.

In his operating theatre just behind the Mareth Line then was consultant surgeon, Colonel James Eastwood RAMC. Nurses working with him remember how one day he performed seventeen operations. Then he visited every patient in the building battered by shells and machine-gun fire; at dusk, he accepted an invitation to knock a tennis ball about on the desert sand. He made two or three strokes and then lay down. Doctors asked what was wrong, but Colonel Jimmy was already dead.

Unknown to most of his colleagues he had been suffering from a painful heart condition, but was determined to carry on with his work. A post-mortem showed how extreme his cardiac condition was. But he was dedicated to doing as much as he could for those who risked their lives every day in driving Rommel into the hands of the Allied First Army advancing from Tunisia.

Nurses had landed there in November 1942 and followed the First Army through the fiercest fighting into the hills of Tebourba, Djedeida and Medjez-el-Bab, Tunisia. Here was not the sun and sand that soldiers had expected from Africa, but cold and mud, and craggy hills and dense scrub, and the Germans attacking with tanks and infantry and complete air superiority.

Nurses followed the infantry with their casualty clearing stations along roads that were bombed from the moment troops moved forward. Those troops and nurses were often wet through, short of kit and exhausted from lack of sleep. But they carried on setting up their units behind those formidable hills as infantry slogged it out with an enemy whose strength was constantly reinforced by German divisions from nearby Sicily. British casualties were heavy. Typical was the situation at Djedeida airfield where the infantry were hit hard. The Hampshire regiment that had landed but one week earlier was sent in to relieve those holding the position in country similar to the broad Hampshire downs. But on the menacing hills overlooking the wood where the Hampshires took their stand was the enemy. The raw soldiers of the Hampshires did not know the ground, only that those who had held it before them were hit grievously hard, as evidenced by the shallow graves nearby, marked with a makeshift cross. Germans waited patiently until the whole battalion was in position below them. Then venomously accurate mortar fire and rapid machine-gun fire plastered their shallow slit trenches.

The Hampshires fixed bayonets, waiting for the German infantry to attack. Time and time again for three days fresh German infantry came into the attack, and each time they were driven back by Bren guns and bayonet, but they answered every challenge with unimaginable ferocity until only a handful of dog-tired Hampshires remained.

Stretcher-bearers, the regimental medical officer and padre worked without rest under the heaviest of fire. The position became hopeless, but rather than surrender they broke into small parties and made for the hills. In that grim action almost the whole battalion of 900 men had been sacrificed. And the way to Tunis was still blocked.

During the next few months of bitterly cold rain, fighting patrols went out night after night, attacks went in to clear Germans from hills whose names are deeply engraved on the memories of those who fought there – those who proudly wear the 1st Army clasp on their

Africa Star ribbon – Tangouche, and the camel-humped Longstop to name but two. (Men and women who served in the North African campaigns were awarded the Africa Star medal. To differentiate between those serving in the 1st Army in Tunisia from those of the 8th in the Western Desert and all qualifying for the Africa Star medal, a clasp showing the figure 1 or 8 was affixed to the medal ribbon.)

### Behind the Line by Estelle Lancaster

The enemy was smashed at Alamein,
A fine battle – or so the general said,
But all we heard were shouts of 'Convoy in!',
And all we saw were wretched, stretchered men,
And all we knew as how the price was paid.

No training steeled us for the scenes were saw,
So pitiful: the splintered bones, the shreds,
The gaping holes in backs and chests and heads,
Poor roasted tankmen, blackened bleeding raw,

With arms torn off or missing half a face,
They bore their suffering with fortitude,
Expressing only warmest gratitude,
And wonder at finding us in that far place.

A woman's presence close behind the line,
Her gentle touch, her smile, her soothing voice,
Was Heaven to those mutilated boys;
Incredulously shadowed eyes would shine.

Distressed and yet unwilling to complain,
They waited whilst we swiftly did our best
To save and comfort first the very worst,
Washing, changing dressings, easing pain.

Row upon row of casualties to tend,
And so few hands to transfuse blood to mend
The broken bodies, plaster splintered limbs,
Inject the morphine, bind the massive wounds.

I remember, while the hours flew,
How one young patient called me from my round

To ask politely if I knew
That he had not been washed, lest we forget.

I reassured: 'Quite soon, but not just yet.
These others need attention urgently,'
'I understand,' he said 'don't worry about me.'
Such humbleness, such equanimity.

Though covered with rough blankets, blood caked, sore,
The quiet acceptance, selfless bravery,
Of British troops would touch us to the core
And banish every trace of weariness.

When all were in clean sheets and wounds were dressed,
Then sisters could be spared to take a nap.
But calls soon broke the deep sleep to wake us up,
Resounding through the compound: 'Convoy in!'
And so our duty would again begin.[11]

# 15 A Damned Close-run Thing

'I must admit I missed the excitement of nursing nearer the battle line. But back home in England I saw how the wounded had fared after passing through our hands abroad.'

Sister Freda Barnfather (now Reid)

At daybreak on 10 July 1943, an Allied invasion fleet of 2,500 ships headed for the beaches of Sicily. Following in the convoy's wake were two hospital ships, the *Tarai* and the *Talamba*, with a full complement of nurses on board. German bombers hit the *Talamba*. It sank within fifteen minutes. Sister Maud Johnson, looking after wounded on the ship, went down with her. Another nurse, with a broken leg, was pulled out of the water with other survivors half an hour later.

By Sunday 12 July the British Eighty Army had taken all its immediate objectives, including the greatest prize of all, the key port of Syracuse. At first they suffered few casualties, which were taken off the beaches by hospital ship *Leinster*. Within a few days, though, the sweat-lathered soldiers were battered by the Hermann Goering Grenadiers, dug in on the volcanic slopes of Mount Etna. Towering over 10,000 feet, it overlooked all lines of approach to Messina. Rough grey lava lay everywhere. This was the killing ground over which the Eighth Army had to fight to reach its Sicilian objectives.

Casualties now were heavy. Wounded men, strapped to stretchers slung on each side of sure-footed mules, were carried down rough mountain tracks to jeeps waiting to take them to hospitals on the Catania Plain. Nursing care was again as close to the fighting as possible to give casualties the best possible chance of recovery. Rose Parker still remembers those men:

The smart, sun-tanned young soldiers we'd watched embarking a few days earlier, were brought to us bleached with white dust, their khaki drill filthy, bloody and torn. Their reddened faces sore, glistening with the sweat of pain and the heat of the piercing Sicilian sun. Many of them, so parched with thirst, had eaten too many green, under-ripe grapes and suffered diarrhoea in addition to their wounds. Worse still, many had ignored warnings about going into vineyards sewn with mines, and had a foot blown to bits. Too often a mate who'd tried to bring them out suffered the same fate.

Soon what had appeared to be a comparatively easy campaign turned out to be a desperate and costly business. On 17 August 1943, thirty-eight days after the Allies had landed, Sicily was captured but not the German army. Most of it had escaped over the Straits of Messina to mainland Italy. The easy conquest of Sicily promised by General Montgomery cost the Allies dearly[1] – the British lost 2,721 killed, 2,183 missing, and 7,939 wounded. The American losses were 2,811 killed, 686 missing and 6,471 wounded – but the victory brought about Mussolini's downfall and Italy's surrender.

For a week or two, nurses were able to get on top of their work, gradually evacuating as many patients as possible to free their wards for the next onslaught, the invasion of mainland Italy. There was still a steady stream of malaria patients, and drastic measures were taken to get rid of anophele mosquitoes in areas where troops were concentrated. Wet breeding grounds were sprayed regularly with dichlor-dyphenyl-trichlotethane DDT, before the more alarming hazards to health from the practice were known.

Pathetic patients also brought into hospitals then were young children who had had their hands blown off by diabolical booby traps left by Germans for Allied soldiers. They looked like bars of chocolate but exploded when lifted.

Nevertheless, by the end of August 1943, the pressure of work eased and nurses found opportunities for entertainment and romance. Sister Marjorie Bennett of the British Medical Hospital, Syracuse, recalled enjoyable evenings in Catania's opera house and at dances given in the hospital mess to repay hospitality received from neighbouring units. At once dance she fell in love with an RAF officer stationed in Malta. A few months later she and her handsome flight-lieutenant were married by the hospital chaplain. Patients formed a guard of honour with bedpans and crutches!

The lull in fighting ended before dawn on 3 September 1943 when 600 guns in the hills above Messina opened fire on Italian coastal batteries across the Straits of Messina. It was the beginning of a long and bitter campaign in which every fortified river and ridge had to be taken with appalling costs in casualties.

That hot summer, as Eighth Army troops slogged their way northwards from the toe of Italy, they found every road and river bridge blown up by Germans withdrawing to defensive positions further north. Meanwhile, ships from many Mediterranean ports were heading for Italy, with more troops and nurses of all three services.

Wherever the RAF was operational their nurses were there too, with advanced surgical units and mobile field hospitals working close to the front line. The surgical units comprised one surgeon, one anaesthetist, two nursing sisters and four medical orderlies. These units gave surgical treatment to casualties very soon after being wounded. With such prompt attention many lives were saved that in previous wars would have been lost.

RAF nursing sisters, dressed either in white uniforms and caps when working in buildings or blue battledress and white shirts when under canvas, also held commissioned ranks equivalent to those of the men: matron = squadron leader; senior sister = flight lieutenant; sister = flying officer.

Into the ports on their hospital ships came nursing sisters of the Queen Alexandra's Royal Naval Nursing Service too. At sea and in ports they ran risks of being attacked from the air or from torpedoes. Death by drowning was a hazard they accepted. One one occasion, in May 1944, forty RN nursing sisters were lost at sea. Lists of nurses killed in action appeared regularly in the nursing journals, above what the poet Wilfred Owen called the 'old lie': 'Dulce et decorum est pro patria mori.'

In July 1943 Mr A.V. Alexander, first lord of the admiralty, circulated what he termed 'an unhappily long list of attacks on 19 hospital ships upon which navy and army nurses paid their last debt of duty to their patients'.

From 1943 onwards a shortage of nurses existed in the armed forces, since restrictions on recruitment allowed only newly qualified nurses to join up. Frequently nurses were constantly working under stress with huge numbers of casualties.[2] Nevertheless, those nurses who survived the war now look back on those hectic days with pride and feelings of satisfaction and even enjoyment in working with such wonderful colleagues.

Early that autumn of 1943, VAD (RN) Jessie Fairchild remembers sailing from Malta's ruined grand harbour in the troopship *Escania*, bound for a military hospital in Calabria, in Italy's toe. She was not sorry to be leaving the island that had been so intensively bombed. Indeed, so many of its hospitals had been hit and nurses killed that the islanders had been presented with the George Cross, an award normally given to individuals. Jessie had been nursing in 90th General Military Hospital, Imtarfa, where she encountered some terrible sights. She remembers vividly two young, badly burnt aircrew from a bomber that had crashed in flames. She had nursed them for months.

Their scorched bodies were swathed completely in Vaseline dressings, like Egyptian mummies, with only a narrow gap over their mouths. Every day, Jessie spoonfed them through that gap, put their arms and hands in saline baths and looked after all their personal bodily needs for weeks. At last the day came to take the bandages from their eyes. Other patients across the ward watched anxiously. Would those young men be blind or now be able to see? 'The last dressing came off. They could see! A great cheer went up,'[3] recalled Jessie.

They were fit enough to travel home. A week later the news came that their ship had been torpedoed. Both had gone down with it. 'To this day I mourn them and they will always live in my memory.'

Yes, she was happy to be leaving the besieged island, as were most of the nurses. They felt excited, looking forward to seeing a new country – Italy.

When Jessie reached the hospital at Brindisi she found the nurses working to a steady routine, for the Eighth Army were not then incurring heavy casualties. There was time enough for nurses to relax in their off-duty hours. Unfortunately for them at Brindisi Field Hospital, nurses were not allowed out unless chaperoned by an armed soldier. This was because of an antagonistic Fascist element in the town. Eventually, though, nurses began to defy the regulations and go out on their own. Jessie Fairchild tells an amusing story of the night she and four nurses did step out unescorted.

They headed for the nearest restaurant, but on turning a corner saw two red-capped army policeman on patrol. Fearing the matron's wrath, they took to their heels, dashing down cobbled backstreets and a maze of dark alleys. Local Italians, eager to help damsels in distress, called out for them to come with them. Now they led the race down even narrower passageways until they came to a small coffee shop. Inside they fled, through tables, a steam-filled kitchen, out of the back door and into a trattoria where locals were having supper.

Breathless, excited and laughing we sank onto hard chairs at a small wooden table. After hearing what had happened the owner presented us with a much appreciated bottle of Chianti.

As Italians got used to the new invaders, restrictions were relaxed and nurses were allowed to roam newly occupied towns. We often visited that trattoria and exchanged our rations of Woodbine cigarettes for a plate of spaghetti.[4]

On 9 September 1943 another convoy was approaching the shores of Italy, carrying 100,000 British and 69,000 American troops. They were preparing to assault the beaches of Salerno and blast their way to the vital seaport of Naples. But on the evening before the landings the ship's radio broadcast the great news that Italy had surrendered. Faces that had been tense and strained were now relaxed and happy. No bloody assault landing after all, they thought. Nurses of 59th General Hospital, who had left Gebeit in the Sudan and destined for an early landing experienced the same sense of relief as the assault troops on hearing the news. Some commanders were not so sanguine.

Field-Marshal Kesselring's men had taken over Italian positions on the hills overlooking the beaches. They let the first battalions land without opposition, the German flares hissed into the night sky. Bursts of machine-gun tracer bullets swept across dark beaches. The fiercest, bloodiest battles of World War Two so far had begun – a situation of utter confusion and horror.

In the rough sea off shore, Sister Margaret Jennings and her colleagues waited until dawn before attempting to jump into their assault craft that were bobbing madly against the side of their ship. They had been given just four hours' notice to leave their hospital in Kantara, Egypt, to sail for Salerno. She remembers clearly that night off Salerno's beaches:

Waves rocked our ship all night. I sat on the deck with our doctor and watched the flashes from guns lighting up the whole coast and hills beyond. The terrific noise of shelling and gunfire was frightening and I thought of the soldiers who had already gone ahead into it all. It seemed a terrible waste.

We made our jump into the barges at five o'clock the next morning. As we approached the beach, we saw the debris of battle including the wreck of a German plane. Suddenly and unexpectedly we had become front-line nurses for we were split into smaller groups for Casualty Clearing Stations and Field Dressing Stations. The Army had realised the mobile medical units ensured that medical treatment could be given more effectively as soon after the wounding as possible.

We got into a truck and were driven forward to our location close

behind the forward lines. On the way civilians cheered and threw
bunches of grapes to us. As we passed infantry marching in single
file on the sides of the road they grinned and cheered. Amazed to
see women so far forward.

Nurses who joined Colonel Watts in his forward Casualty Clearing
Station found they were quickly on a conveyor-belt of work, as he
later noted: 'We had a first-class group of sisters and we received five
hundred and twelve casualties in one day. The theatre, installed in a
large classroom, was going full blast and we had to evacuate as many
patients as possible the next day. American nurses were working close
to us too.'[5]

Casualties were carried to the shore and loaded on to special low-
draft boats that went alongside the hospital ship *Leinster* to be
hoisted on to its deck, before setting off for Tunisian hospitals. Not all
hospital ships got back though. All had to risk being bombed, despite
the red crosses painted on their sides and deck. Sister Mary Johnston,
aboard the *Leinster* in the bay, saw the *Newfoundland* hit and sink.
She also witnessed the *St Andrew* picking up survivors in the water,
among whom were nurses who were landed on the beachhead.

Operating under battlefield conditions, surgeons had to make decisions at speed and sometimes use improvised facilities. Instruments
were sterilized in a fish-kettle boiled on a primus stove; hands were
washed thoroughly in a tin basin and then spirit was poured over
them. 'Emergency anaesthesia was achieved by an injection of
pentathol into a vein and ether given on a simple mask. Sometimes
we operated at night by the light of a Tilly lamp worked on the
Primus principle,' recalled Colonel Watts.[6]

For weeks the whole military venture at Salerno seemed hopeless.
Allied infantry could not move forward because German troops held
fortified positions on the hills, and several times they were nearly
pushed back into the sea. Everyone was within range of German
artillery. At last, on 23 September, X Corps forced a passage from
Salerno to Naples. But as Eisenhower later remarked, 'It was a
damned close-run thing!'

With the capture of Naples, Allied nurses took over wards in
Italian hospitals and other buildings. But routine work was difficult.
German rear parties had smashed sewage systems, drained reservoirs,
blown up aqueducts and left time-bombs in public buildings. German
bombers raided Naples almost every night. British hospitals were hit
and nurses killed. Sister Jennings, up from Salerno, joined Number 92
General Hospital just before bombs wrecked one ward. 'One of our

nurses was killed and another seriously injured. They had not been able to get to cover before the first shower of bombs rained down. Naples was a tempting target with troopships packing the port.'

In December 1943, on the Adriatic side of Italy, Allied divisions were being decimated on the slopes of Monte Cassino. Sister Michelle Higgs had never before seen as many mutilated casualties as streamed into her casualty clearing station below that impregnable fortress on the Gustav Line.

It was on Christmas Day 1943 when nurses heard with some trepidation President Roosevelt broadcast to the Allies. He warned that 'the war is now reaching the stage when we shall have to look forward to large casualty lists – dead, wounded and missing. War entails just that. There is no easy road to victory. And the end is not yet in sight.'

There seemed to be no way of avoiding further heavy casualties at Monte Cassino except by simply holding the line. This tactic at least had the benefit of keeping the German armies occupied until the Second Front was opened in Normandy. But Churchill had other ideas. Convalescing from a chest infection in the luxury of his villa at Marakesh, he was in the capable hands of 29-year-old QA Sister Elizabeth Lavinia Clarke, a pitman's daughter from Chopwell, County Durham. She had been flown with all secrecy from her hospital in Egypt to nurse him back to health. In the peace of his Marakesh residence, Churchill thought the Allies should by-pass Cassino by making an assault landing north of the Gustav Line.

So it was that on 21 January 1944, 242 ships took a massive Allied force to the beaches of Anzio thirty-five miles south of Rome. The objective was to cut off and capture the entire German Tenth Army manning the Gustav Line.

But, once again, the Germans were a step ahead, with troops in readiness. Indecisive leadership and arguments amongst Allied generals resulted in soldiers and nurses being stranded for four months on a beachhead constantly under artillery fire.

Nurses on the beachhead had to ignore shrapnel whizzing through the canvas covering weapon pits that had been turned into operating theatres and dressing stations. They slept in slit trenches that filled with mud from January until March. Trapped on the Anzio beachhead the Allies could make no progress. Then on 18 May Monte Cassino was captured and Allied troops drove northwards to link up with the Anzio beachhead. Days later, 150,000 Allied soldiers broke out of the perimeter and pursued the retreating Germans. The Allies entered Rome on 4 June 1944.

'How magnificently your troops have fought,' Churchill telegraphed to Roosevelt. But British newspapers had little space for news of that success in Italy. Two days after the Americans entered Rome, the Allies invaded Normandy: 'D-Day!'

Senior VAD Joyce Dury, then Saunders, stationed at HMS *Impregnable*, above Devonport dockyard, saw part of that invasion flotilla gathering.

> Small craft had been anchoring in 'threes' up the creek for weeks, waiting. There was no shore leave. On the night of June 6th 1944 this changed. They were now side by side in single file ready to peel off for sea. As I looked down on this historic phenomenon I wondered how many of these small craft would survive. Next morning, the seventh, the creek was empty. It was an eerie feeling. We knew it had begun.

Among that invasion flotilla were hospital ships and carriers with their complement of nurses. More Navy, Army and Air Force nurses of mobile field hospitals, casualty clearing stations and tented base hospitals were ready for the crossing. Sister Iris Ogilvie, of the Princess Mary's RAF Nursing Service, sailed in a tank landing ship.

> Everything went so smoothly. A meal was ready just after we sailed. We joined a queue. A dollop of stew and potatoes in one mess tin and rice pudding in another. We dozed and woke at dawn to see a smoky haze over the coast ahead. A tremendous banging jolted us all. Alongside us a cruiser pounded enemy strongpoints. A short time later the ship shuddered to a stop. The front ramp dropped and tanks squealed and clattered down the ramp onto the beach. Then came our turn. We jogged down the metal ramp onto Juno/Red Beach, Courseulles-sur-Mer. In the half light we followed shady figures up the beach. Our nurses kept together. No one knew where our assembly point was. 'Get down' someone shouted. Deafening explosions shook the ground near us. Great red balls seemed to come straight at me. A soldier ran up shouting our unit number. He led us to our Mobile Hospital.
>
> Troop Carrying Vehicles took us away. We stopped and immediately everybody was working, erecting tents, unpacking equipment as if on a training exercise. Everything worked so well. Later the next day we received our first casualties.

Waiting in a tank landing ship just off shore was Sister Marie Sedman of Number 75 Field Hospital:

Things had not gone according to plan for us. The infantry had not taken their first objectives and we couldn't go ashore until the site for our hospital had been taken. Our ship zigzagged along the coast for two days. Most of us were sea-sick. When eventually we landed on the beach, eight of us were detailed for Number 2 Field Dressing Station at Courseulles, the rest of the nurses joined Number 81 British General Hospital. Nothing in our training could have prepared us for the sudden shock of being part of such a bloody scene. But the strict discipline of our training did help us to get on with the job. The worst, I found, were the burnt tank crews. So little was left of their arms, just like charred sticks.

As soon as those first hospitals were operational, convoys of wounded arrived by the hundred. After wounds were dressed, beds had to be emptied as soon as possible to make way for the next convoy. At times hospitals acted as Casualty Clearing Stations, with patients being in and out again within forty-eight hours. One hospital took 1048 cases in one day and a Sister said some of her beds had been filled and emptied three times in forty eight hours.[7]

Usually a triage team was set up to separate the wounded on arrival into two main classes: the more serious cases requiring immediate attention and others who could wait for operative treatment. There was a third section of terribly wounded men for whom little could be done other than easing pain and making them as comfortable as possible until they died.

For those not evacuated on hospital ships there was a quicker means of getting back to Britain – by air direct to RAF Hospital Wroughton, Wiltshire. Rosemary Gannon of the WAAF remembers how their reception team was assembled in great secrecy in late May 1944 and confined to camp. The wing commander said: 'It's all about to happen. When the hooter sounds go immediately to your designated operations theatre to receive the severely wounded.'

When Myra Roberts, Lydia Alford and Edna Birkbeck of the WAAF medical section volunteered for the duty of flying nursing attendant they never for a moment realized how soon they would be bouncing over makeshift runways on French beaches in a Dakota aircraft, leaping out and then packing stretchers of bleeding men into the fuselage as fast as possible. 'Rarely had we time for a "comfort break" before we took off again. Even then we had to find the nearest bush.'

Field surgical units were set up close to the front line. They were so effective that the deputy director of medical services reported that they could perform top quality surgery and almost any operation within six hours, consequently reducing considerably the risks of septic wounds.[8]

Blood transfusion facilities were also available. Refrigerated trucks, sometimes called 'vampire vans' went round units, topping up supplies. Whole blood was used, and sometimes as a temporary measure, plasma. Nurses in forward areas helped with the transfusions for resuscitation, shock therapy and the preparation of patients to withstand surgery.[9]

The sheer physical demands of nursing, the concentration required and the absolute horror of dealing with badly wounded men put great emotional strain on all nurses. Yet, unfailingly, they stood up to that drain on their stock of emotional energy.

> Occasionally, I confess, I just had to leave the ward hurriedly with tears brimming in my eyes at seeing so many disfigured and maimed young lads that I couldn't trust myself to speak [recalled Marie Floyd Norris (then Sedman)], but usually we all managed to mask our innermost feelings. It was the only way. That and just getting on with jobs to be done.
>
> Of all the terrible wounds I remember most of all the burns. Once I saw a squadron of tanks going up the line past our hospital. We waved to them and it was not long before they were back in our wards with fifth and sixth degree burns. They had to be treated with so much care so that they were kept warm yet with nothing really touching their burnt bodies. We used cradles to keep them warm yet free from anything actually touching the burns. Limbs were floated in a saline filled bag. All had liberal doses of morphia.

By the time troops reached the Rhine in March 1945 another kind of wound became increasingly prevalent: the wounded mind. Many soldiers had seen years of active service by that time and were war weary. They had had enough. Enough anxiety, enough of seeing their mates killed, enough of being told to get ready for just one more action. In medical jargon they were suffering from 'anxiety states' or 'disturbed neurosis'. Soldiers called it being 'bomb happy'. Nurses and medical officers soon became familiar with the condition.

Indeed, nurses themselves suffered. One matron advised nurses who had reached the end of their tether to get involved with trivial tasks for a short while until they felt in control again. In time, some doctors and nurses were driven to extreme and tragic actions. A medical officer serving with Number 75 British General Hospital became so disturbed dealing with 2,400 admissions in eleven days that he seized a scalpel, slashed both brachial arteries and shot himself.[10]

Fortunately for soldiers by 1944, the high command and medical officers recognized that fit young men could become seriously mentally disturbed by seeing friends they had trained with in Britain having their heads or legs blown off, and it was better to take action before men became too ill. In Italy, for example, special 'rest and recuperation' camps took front-line soldiers for a week's leave. They could rest, swim, be entertained by visiting artists or even go to see *Madama Butterly* at the nearby Teatro di San Carlo, in Naples.

Casualties who were brought to hospitals suffering from battle fatigue were usually washed, put into clean pyjamas, sometimes given a mild dose of Pentothal and allowed to rest for a few days. After physical rehabilitation and occupational therapy many of them could return to their units. In 1944 the 32nd General Hospital was sent to Normandy for this specific duty.

Sadly some patients never responded to treatment. Many hospitals had tales to tell of suicides, through wrists cut with razor blades, or an overdose of drugs somehow saved or stolen.

Seeing friends mutilated beyond recognition eventually became too much for some front-line soldiers and even for nurses. Marie Sedman's experience with severe facial injuries came when she took charge of a ward in a maxillo-facial unit in Number 8 Medical Hospital in Brussels:

Some men had parts of their faces blown away by high explosive shells. Each individual was different. Each coped with excruciating pain in his own way. One day a grey-haired gentleman in a black suit came into the ward and talked to soldiers. I didn't know until the Commanding Officer came into my ward later that evening and told me the visitor was Sir Harold Gillies from St Mary's Hospital, Sidcup, who was the top specialist in plastic surgery in the First World War too. What delighted the C.O., was that Sir Harold said he had never seen men with such severe burns so well looked after.

We'd been told that we should look badly disfigured men in the eyes when talking to them, if they had any, and try not to let our feelings show on our faces. We had German casualties as well as Allied and one day I was given an unforgettable token of their gratitude which I have kept to this day. The incident happened whilst I was dressing wounds at the end of the ward and one of the German patients, blinded in both eyes, had got out of bed in an attempt to feel his way to the lavatory. The poor chap could not make it in time and made a mess on the floor. I didn't see what happened next but patients soon told me. A British orderly came into the ward, saw the mess on the floor and shouted at the German to clean it up. I saw the German trying to do his best with a mop and took it from him and finished the job myself. I reprimanded the orderly and when I came back into the ward after washing my hands one of the German patients who spoke English came to me with something wrapped in tissue paper. 'We all want you to have this, Sister,' he said. I opened it and saw the medal. 'It's the Iron Cross,' said the German. 'No, no, I can't take this. It's too precious for you,' I said. He took hold of my hands, closed them round the little tissue-paper parcel and turned me to face the German patients in their beds. 'Look,' he said, 'We all want you to have it.' They were all nodding and smiling. I was just too full to say anything more. Tears welled in my eyes, I brushed a hand over my face and walked away.[11]

By the middle of March 1945 the German army in north-west Europe began their bitter retreat, their route marked by purple frozen dead bodies. On Sunday, 29 April, the 15th Scottish Division crossed the Elbe and broke through to Hamburg and Lübeck before the Russians. Now it was virtually over.

Of the final stages of the war in Europe there is no need to go into further detail except to remind the reader that though the end came quickly, it came only through tremendous personal sacrifice to the last day. On 4 May 1945 the war against Germany was over. Yet to be concluded was that with Japan.

War in the Far East began for nurses on 7 December 1941 when Japanese bombers hit Hong Kong and the Royal Naval hospital where superintending sister, Miss Olga Frankin, had already made contingency arrangements for patients' safety by emptying the upper wards. The next day low-flying Japanese fighter bombers wrecked the top floor of the hospital and machine-gunned wildly all about the hospital. They came in the evening, too, while surgeons were amputating legs and arms by candlelight. Worse was to come.

On 18 December Japanese infantry broke through the weak British defences, bayoneting any soldier still standing. Then crazed by victory and alcohol, they battered the doors of the hospital, slaughtered fifty-six patients in their beds and raped nurses.[12]

At that time, too, Japanese troops were advancing down the Malayan peninsula and on to Singapore. There again, despite huge red crosses painted on all hospital buildings and on the square, Japanese pilots dive-bombed and machine-gunned them. Immediately the air-raid alarm sounded, nursing sisters moved patients on the ground floor under their beds and patients from top floors joined them. Quickly the situation got worse. Japanese artillery shelled all buildings, killing doctors and nurses.

Numbers 17 and 20 combined general hospitals were wrecked by bombs. Sisters hurried to the docks as machine-gun bullets ricocheted around them. The blazing docks already looked like a shambles, but evacuation ships were waiting. The *Empire Star* was already packed with more than 2,000 army and air force troops, as well as Australian sisters and VADs, but a few more squeezed aboard. They sailed next morning. Despite the constant air raids some nurses managed to snatch a few hours' sleep in the hold. These were the lucky nurses who reached Batavia safely.

Many of the fifty sisters who left Singapore just one day later in the ss *Kuala* lost their lives when the ship was bombed and sank immediately. Among those drowned or killed by the explosions were the principal matron of Alexandra hospital, Miss Jones, and matron of Number 1 Malayan Hospital, Miss West and matrons from No. 17 and 20 Combined General Hospitals a Miss Russel and Miss Coward. Other nurses desperately clinging to floating debris in the sea were machine-gunned and bombed yet again. A swift current carried a few survivors to various small islands. Twenty-three of them who eventually landed on the small island of Banka were ordered by Japanese soldiers to wade back into the sea. They realized what was going to happen to them and had just reached a depth of waist height, when their matron, Irene Drummond, called out to them: 'Chin up girls. I'm proud of you and I love you all.' At that point the Japanese machine-guns fired. All died except one who faked death and later told what happened to a war crimes tribunal in Tokyo:

> I was towards the end of the line and a bullet got me in the left loin and went straight through. The force knocked me over into the water and I lay there. The waves brought me back to the edge of the water. I lay there, not moving for ten minutes. Then I sat up slowly. There was no sign of anybody. I got up and went into the jungle and lay down. I slept or was unconscious for two days.[13]

When she came round she found fresh water and bathed her wounds. Then she went in search of food in a nearby Indonesian village. After about twelve days she gave herself up to a Japanese officer. She spent the next three-and-a-half years moving from one squalid prison camp to another. She confided her story to Colonel Modein of the British army, who told her to keep her story secret otherwise the Japanese would surely kill her. In November 1946, still recovering from her ordeal, she gave evidence at the war crimes tribunal. She learnt later that the officer who had ordered the shooting of the nurses had committed suicide rather than face justice.

In 1993 Vivian Bullwinkel returned to the beach on Banka Island to unveil a memorial to the nurses who had died there. She donated her diaries and the uniform she was wearing when she was shot, complete with bullet holes, to the Australian War Memorial's permanent collection.

She died aged 84, when this chapter was being written, in July 2000.

Nurses who landed on Sumatra were captured by the Japanese and spent the rest of the war as prisoners. Nurses in internment camps were subjected to humiliating tasks, given starvation rations, and for no apparent reason sentenced to occasional bouts of imprisonment in cells where they slept on stone flags without a blanket.

It is not possible here, for lack of space, to detail the appalling experiences endured with such fortitude by these nurses for the rest of the war. Accounts of the atrocities perpetrated against nurses by Japanese soldiers, of them being raped, bayoneted and shot in cold blood, should be read in factual detail in the appropriate official reports and in eye-witness accounts.

In Britain relatives of those nurses stationed in the Far East were horrified to hear what was happening to their loved ones in a short catalogue of Japanese atrocities given to Members of the House of Commons on 10 March 1942 by foreign secretary Anthony Eden.

In the early summer of 1945, though, formidable retribution for the Japanese was well on the way. The Fourteenth Army in Burma was pushing back Japanese forces across the Irrawaddy with the last, the greatest and least publicized of all the Allied victories of the Second World War. In Kohima, Imphal and beyond the Japanese, fighting with fanatical ferocity, suffered appalling losses. Nurses were close to the front working in wards made from bamboo.

At the same time an even bigger force of American infantry and marines was advancing beyond Okinawa and Luzon in bloody battles, fighting sometimes hand to hand.

On 9 March, 278 B29 bombers of the United States Air Force devastated Tokyo with incendiaries. All major Japanese cities, Osaka, Kobe and Nagoya, suffered the same devastation. Japanese morale sank. Everyone now saw that unconditional surrender was unavoidable.

On 20 June Emperor Hirohito asked the Soviet Union to negotiate peace to stop the bloodshed, but the United States was determined to force the Japanese to their knees. To convince the emperor an atomic bomb was dropped on Hiroshima on 6 August 1945, killing 80,000 people. Two days later, Stalin declared war on Japan. Nagasaki was bombed the next day, and on 2 September 1945 Japan representatives signed the instrument of surrender on US battleship *Missouri*.

The war was over, but Stalin's declaration of war against Japan entitled him to take an active role in Far Eastern affairs.

In the terms of surrender, Japan lost control of Korea, which it had governed since 1910. It was divided in two parts, the north going to the Communists and the south to a government claiming to be democratic. Russia immediately occupied the area north of the 38th parallel and established a Communist government. The division of Korea in 1945 was a recipe for disaster. It would lead, in less than five years, to the Korean War.

# 16 When the Cold War Became Hot

'One of Britain's most successful contributions to the United Nations' effort in the Korean War has been HM Hospital Ship *Maine*.'[1]

Lord Fraser of North Cape, First Sea Lord, 1950

Before dawn on the wet morning of 25 June 1950, just five years after the end of the Second World War, Russian-backed North Korean forces launched a blitzkrieg-style attack on American-protected South Korea. First came a heavy artillery barrage, which served as a declaration of war, then over 150 Russian-built T-34 tanks drove across the 38th parallel, striking towards the South Korean capital, Seoul, and to major ports on the east and west coasts of the Korean peninsula.

The country, ruled by Japan since 1910, had been divided into two halves at the 38th parallel, when Japan was defeated in 1945. The Soviet Union occupied the northern half and the United States moved into the southern to curtail the spread of Communism.

In June 1950, North Korea attempted to reunify the country by invading the South. The United States was committed to 'containment', a 'Cold War' with the Soviet Union aimed at preventing Communism from controlling nations beyond where it already held sway. Already Eastern Europe was under Soviet control, Berlin had been blockaded by Russian troops, and Communists had taken over Czechoslovakia. Western Europe was under threat. In view of such threats, the United States had, in April 1950, approved the rearmament of West Germany.

When North Korea's army crossed the 38th parallel, President Truman sent American troops to Korea and called upon the United Nations to send peace-keeping troops to the area in addition. The UN

Security Council authorized the organization of a UN force comprising troops, including nurses, from twenty-two nations, in order to maintain an independent South Korea. The bulk of the force came from the United States.

The North's massive invasion force of 25 June 1950 took the ill-equipped South Korean army completely off guard. Weekend-leave passes had been issued to officers of the South Korean Army. Soldiers, woken from sleep by shellfire, panicked and fled. Gull-winged *Stormovick* dive-bombers, demoralized fleeing soldiers before they had time to recover from the first shelling. Retreat turned into a panic-driven rout, except for a few heroic South Korean soldiers who stuffed their shirts with explosives and threw themselves under North Korean tanks. But there was a shortage of suicide volunteers.

At short notice, the commander-in-chief Far East, General MacArthur, sent two US infantry divisions to man front-line defences in Korea. These men had no time in training to get psychologically or physically fit to face the savage combat conditions ahead.

Imagine their feelings. They had been living almost as civilians with servants in Japan, when they were suddenly dumped into a fearsome war. They were shocked on arrival at the port of Pusan to see train-loads of bloodstained South Korean soldiers being lifted on to ambulances. A second morale-sagging shock came as they drove north and passed truckloads of South Korean soldiers fleeing in the opposite direction.

During their first two weeks in the front line, the raw GI recruits had no weapons capable of stopping the North Korean tanks. Cynically they joked that 'shortages were all the army had in abundance'. They suffered frightful casualties in hellish heat and hostile hilly scrubland, or quagmires of paddy fields. These conditions would have taxed to the limit even the fittest, battle-seasoned soldiers.

Sister Gillian Hall (later McNair), QARANC – the QAIMNS became part of the British army on 1 February 1949 – first saw the country through a small window in an old Dakota aircraft. 'We were sitting in a bare fuselage with long canvas seating on each side of the plane. We took off at five in the morning and in the bright sunshine I could see snatches of a sparse, barren land, craggy hills with a jigsaw of paddy fields in between.'[2]

It was difficult terrain to defend against overwhelming odds. By the end of July 1950, three American divisions, making up the American Eighth Army under General Walton Walker, fell back to the Pusan corner of Korea. This was to be a fortress held at all costs. To the south of this 4,000-square mile Pusan redoubt was the sea; the fortress was therefore safe from attack, since US and Royal Navy warships controlled Korean waters. Along the eighty miles of its western front was the Naktong River, which served as a good defensive moat. The northern front was ideally suited for defence, with high mountains overlooking all approaches. Within this area, a good network of roads ensured facilities for transporting troops from one threatened area to another.

Into this fortress trickled the military contributions made by UN countries. From Britain came two brigades, more than half of them national servicemen. Others were regulars and Z reservists, who had left the army after the Second World War, resumed civilian jobs, married and had children. Suddenly they were called back for active service. By the end of August 1950 a force of 40,000 had sailed for Korea from Britain.

A similar mixture of troops for the UN force in the Pusan perimeter, came from Belgium, France, Turkey, Australia, the Netherlands, the Philippines and, surprisingly, Luxembourg. Eventually twenty-two nations took part. Their forces arrived at Pusan and settled in for a siege, General Walker switching them to whichever part of the line was attacked.

Obviously, the Pusan redoubt was not then a place for nurses, nor hospitals. Out of a small medical corps that did go to Pusan in the early days, two RAMC officers were killed and the unit pulled out. Nurses were, nevertheless, near enough in their hospital ship to give swift help. As soon as the United States intervened in Korea, Britain's new socialist prime minister, Clement Attlee, dispatched the Royal Navy's Far Eastern Fleet, with its hospital ship, *Maine*, to join the US Pacific Fleet.

Consequently British nurses were soon in action caring for casualties on the 26-year-old *Maine*. The ship had a curious military history. It had served as an Italian troopship called *Leonardo da Vinci*, then after its capture by the British in 1942, it was used as a British army trooper *Empire Clyde*, to ferry home former prisoners of war from the Far East. Finally, after a refit, it had gone into service with the Royal Navy as HMHS *Maine II*.

Sister (later Matron) Ruth Stone of the QARNNS recalled how the *Maine* was fully ready for action with a full complement of staff: one principal medical officer, four medical officers, one dental officer, one matron, four nursing sisters, six naval VADs, one wardmaster and thirty sick-berth staff plus 100 Maltese deckhands – not forgetting Thomas, the dignified black-and-white ship's cat.

Quite by chance in June 1950, the *Maine* was on manoeuvres with a large detachment of US carriers and battleships as part of a joint naval exercise, when the Korean emergency arose. *Maine* was put at the disposal of the American admiral.

'For several weeks,' wrote Ruth Stone, 'the *Maine* was the only ship on the scene of operations. In one month we made eight trips between Pusan and Japan evacuating a total of 1849 casualties, nearly all of them American soldiers.'[3]

As soon as the *Maine* docked at Pusan nurses were busy loading casualties to be taken to the base hospital across the Korean Straits and through the narrow Shimonoseki channel to Japan. Loading a full complement of casualties took twelve hours, but even before the ship sailed, the surgeons were often already operating on the critically wounded. They continued surgery throughout the voyage, provided the sea was calm. In stormy weather, it was too dangerous to attempt operations. Amputations were frequent because of gangrene setting in quickly. Wounds were typically contaminated by soil which had been heavily fertilized with human excrement. As soon as surgeons finished an operation, patients were labelled on their wrists.

Surgeons, theatre sisters and ward sisters barely had time to take even a cup of tea or a sandwich on those trips between Pusan and Japan. Miss Barbara Nockholds, who had survived the devastating raids on the Royal Naval Hospital, Bighi, during the height of the blitz on Malta in 1941, was on the *Maine* on those hectic journeys as a RN nursing sister. She stepped in to relieve theatre sisters or ward sisters below deck whenever she felt relief was needed; she herself seemed to have inexhaustible supplies of energy. So impressed was *Daily Mail* war correspondent, Ralph Izzard, he was moved to report: 'She is a rare, inspiring, imperturbable and supremely capable woman who never seems to tire.'

Like all good managers, she led from the front. In the not-too-distant future she would become matron-in-chief of the QARNNS. Her presence in those wards below deck was always appreciated by the hundred or so sweating, pain-ridden soldiers lying in temperature ranging from 90 to 116°F. It was especially hot in those 'water-line' wards, because regulations required portholes to be fully closed when at sea. Patients, however, knew their plight was not forgotten when they saw their matron mopping her brow as she frequently made the rounds of all the cots. Little could be done about the heat except to have a plentiful supply of lime juice and water brought round to patients. Jugs of it were placed at points where walking wounded could serve it to their less fortunate comrades.

Sister Ruth Stone remembers, too, that 'battle-fatigued patients in that Dante's Inferno were sedated to spite the noise of the all too near ship's engines below'. It was not surprising that many of those raw American infantrymen were suffering from battle fatigue even though they had been in action but a short time. In that dismal country of Korea, with shabby sprawling towns – 'not one of which is worth fighting for', wrote war correspondent James Cameron – there was enough to sicken even the most hardened veteran soldiers.

In the Pusan pocket, there were not enough troops to hold the front adequately. Troop movements, especially those up and down the craggy hills on the northern front, were particularly exhausting, especially in bad weather. When the sun was not scorching soldiers red raw, pouring rain drenched their clothes and turned the dusty countryside into a quagmire. And all the time it was one near-defeat after another as they advanced and retreated across ground that stank to high heaven with the human excrement used for manure and the unburied dead lying abandoned to the flies.

So many men were getting killed and wounded that one exasperated lieutenant screamed hysterically at journalist Marguerite Higgins: 'Are you correspondents telling people back home the truth?' He asked if they were revealing that only three men out of his platoon of twenty had survived and that it was an 'utterly useless war'.[4]

All too many of those green American troops had the same experiences to tell their nurses. They had sailed from Japan with the idea that 'they'd be a week in Korea to settle the gook thing', but had quickly learnt the reality of their predicament as soon as the 'gooks' attacked in their T-34 tanks with 75 mm cannon; all the GIs had to defend themselves with were weapons last used in a war five years earlier.

Not surprisingly, war in that hostile terrain and the way they had been thrown into the thick of it with so little preparation was a lot to expect from those young soldiers. On top of the horrors at the front they encountered other sickening ones, such as the bodies of US soldiers, murdered in cold blood with their hands wired behind their backs. To a *Yorkshire Post* war correspondent one GI said bitterly: 'I'll fight for my country but I'll be damned if I see why I'm fighting for this hellhole.'[5]

It was indeed such a hellhole that war correspondents were prevented from sending back the full story to their newspapers. Here, after all, were American and British troops fighting to preserve the government of Syngman Rhee, where hundreds of innocent citizens were murdered; where corruption flourished; where police black-mailed citizens, threatening to denounce them as communists for execution without trial; where police set up brothels with destitute refugee girls, and protected distillers of highly dangerous liquor concocted for Allied troops.

Reuters correspondent John Colless saw police shoot fifty-six civilians as 'communist political prisoners' alongside Sarwin railway station and then watched American troops give first aid to those who had not died outright. Peter Webb of United Press, travelling with 20th British Brigade, reported how 'armed South Korean military police kept United Nations troops back whilst their firing squad executed a batch of prisoners amongst whom were women and children'.

At last one war correspondent could no longer stand by and let the murders go on. Australian Alan Dower saw a firing squad forming up in front of a line of men, women carrying babies and children kneeling in front of a trench into which they were to fall and be buried. He stormed into the prison governor's office overlooking the scene, pointed his carbine at the governor sitting behind his desk, and said 'If those machine guns fire I'll shoot you between the eyes.' He extracted a promise that the prisoners would be spared, under the threat that if they were not he, Dower, would personally come and shoot the governor himself.[6]

Angry war correspondents, sickened by the terrible actions done in the name of the so-called democratic southern government sheltering behind the name of the United Nations, complained to the commander-in-chief, General Douglas MacArthur. But to little avail. The vain general, who had ordered a complete news blackout in December 1944 when events were not going well for his command, responded to the complaints of the war correspondents in 1950 in the same way. He imposed full military censorship on all news broadcasts and photographs.

Correspondents were forbidden to make any criticism of the Allied conduct of the war or 'any derogatory comment about UN troops'. And to make sure his orders were obeyed he promised that any correspondent dispatching uncensored reports would be court-martialled. He had already expelled seventeen war correspondents from Japan for criticizing his policies.

And MacArthur had more than South Korean atrocities to hide. He did his best, for example, to hush up the awful casualties that Sister Ruth Stone and her colleagues loaded on to the *Maine* in the last week of September 1950:

I can clearly remember the hectic activity alongside the quays of dusty Pusan harbour, the fleets of ambulances from the ambulance

trains carrying wounded of the Argyll and Sutherland Highlanders
and the 1st Battalion the Middlesex Regiment, who had been badly
burnt from wrongly aimed napalm air attack. The ambulances in the
docks weaved their way through stacks of yellow-ringed American
napalm bombs. At the bottom of our gangway, the Senior Medical
Officer and Wardmaster assessed the gravity of each patient's condition and allocated him to an appropriate ward. The dangerously and
seriously wounded were directed to the one and only ward with air
conditioning: less critically injured to those wards adjacent, and the
walking wounded to the waterline wards, a deck below.

At the other end of the ship, and a deck above, the critically
injured were amassed; the dying in free swinging cots to lessen the
effects of the ship's pitching.

Gradually the news came out of what had happened to those unfor-
tunate victims of the 'wrongly aimed' air attack. At dawn on Friday, 22
September 1950, the Argyll and Sutherland Highlanders had moved
off, laden with packs, rifles and grenades, mortars, mortar shells and
the usual digging-in gear that the 'poor bloody infantry' carried into
battle. They trudged steadily through paddy fields and up hills to take
up positions on the American division's left flank of the front line. The
American General Walker was in command of all troops.

They were to assault and capture Hill 282. By nightfall they dug in
their positions at the base of the hill. At four o'clock the next morning they were roused, and began the steady climb up the hill. It got
lighter by the minute. The summit could just be seen when enemy
automatics and mortars opened fire. The Highlanders rushed the
position and by nine that morning had taken possession of enemy
weapon pits. Some managed to open a tin of bully beef, warm and
mushy. Others did not have time.

The enemy counter-attacked with a shower of mortar bombs
preceding a barrage of artillery shells. Argyll casualties mounted
rapidly. American field guns could not give supporting fire. They were
'needed elsewhere'. North Koreans rushed the Argyll's positions.
They were repelled. Again the Highlanders suffered heavy casualties
and now were so short of ammunition they had to rob the dead for
their clips of rounds. Still no artillery support came. An air strike was
offered. The Argylls put out recognition strips. North Koreans,
already wise to US air strikes, cunningly put out matching recognition
strips too (or so it was later claimed in the Court of Enquiry).

From the US airfield, eager pilots in their P51 Mustangs, bombed
up and with cannons loaded, took off. The Argylls saw them coming,

high in the sky. Moments later they were swooping down, cannons chattering, sending streams of white tracer 20 mm shells into the Argyll slit trenches! They flicked away, flew round once and then levelled out to let go their lethal jellied petrol firebombs, later known to the world as napalm. Bright orange and red flames roared across the hill-top positions like an enormous blowtorch. Men, blackened and shrunken creatures, screamed in agony. Then the planes were gone, leaving a horrendous scene of charred men, dead and dying.

The nearest war correspondent to the scene, Rene Cutforth, described how he saw the napalm canisters drop slowly to earth and burst on impact into a scorching flame. He was shocked by the searing flame of their impact, the rush of intense heat and temperature and then by what he described as 'the reassuring smell of roast pork, for that's what a napalmed human being smells like'.[7]

Reports sent back to Britain were repressed on the grounds that 'they would give aid and comfort to the enemy'.

There was so much that those war correspondents wanted to tell about conditions men and nurses were then facing. Ruth Stone remembered how war correspondent Randolph Churchill, son of the former prime minister, sailed on the *Maine*. 'He wrote a blistering report on the inadequacy of the resources of the *Maine* during the war into which it had been tossed.' Nevertheless, the *Maine* was most effective in saving lives, as Ruth later wrote:

> The sea voyage to Japan could be a calm two-day trip but typhoons could add five days to the normal transit time. Surgeons operated whenever they could. It was generally accepted that those with penetrating abdominal wounds should have colostomies; all chest wounds should be treated with some form of under-water seal drainage, and head injuries, especially of the neck region, should undergo a tracheotomy operation.

One time-consuming but very important duty carried out during the voyage was the administration of an intra-muscular injection of penicillin every morning and evening. At that time penicillin was prepared in a suspension of beeswax, which was difficult to draw up speedily into a syringe. Fortunately for the hard-pressed nurses on the hospital ship, the task of giving penicillin injections was taken over by the dental officer and his assistant, who, said Ruth, 'toiled from bed to bed, and each evening they began all over again. This they somehow achieved in addition to attending to intricate jaw and facial reconstructions which presented themselves on each trip.'

It came as a shock to nurses in the Korean War, just as it had in the Second World War, to find maggots inside wounds, under scalps and even in the first colostomy dressings, before they got patients into the care of the base hospitals in Japan. There, David Oates, a national serviceman who was part of a surgical team at the British Commonwealth general hospital at Kure, recalled his surprise when he removed plaster of Paris from a leg and found maggots everywhere. 'But they had cleaned the wound well! Fortunately the patient was anaesthetised and he was spared the shock.'

Throughout July and August 1950 casualties poured into those base hospitals as North Koreans attacked the Pusan Perimeter ferociously. But during those months more men and weaponry arrived from the United States. By the end of August 1950, the defenders had more men and guns than the North Koreans. They also had 500 medium and heavy tanks. Pusan was safe and it looked as though the Korean War had reached a stalemate. Then General MacArthur withdrew the Marines.

They were to train for an amphibious landing further up the coast, near the key city of Seoul. That assault landing, planned for Inchon, broke all the rules for a successful amphibious operation. The high and low tides there span up to thirty-two feet, and low tide leaves nothing behind but mudflats, preventing further reinforcements or an escape route until the next high tide. Even with a high tide the marines would have to climb ladders to get over the twelve-foot sea wall.

The joint chiefs of staff tried to dissuade MacArthur from his plan. They failed. MacArthur got his way. He assembled an invasion force of 70,000 men. To everyone's surprise, even MacArthur's, the landing succeeded. On 27 September, just over three months after the war started, the South Korean capital city, Seoul, was retaken. The North Korean army was no longer an effective fighting force. Or so it seemed.

The United Nations had achieved their aims: they had cleared the North Korean army from the South and shown emphatically that they would not tolerate communist attempts to expand their rule. And that could well have been the end of the Korean War. No more dead and mutilated men. But . . . there were many 'buts'.

'But' there was no stopping the victorious MacArthur. 'But' North Korea with Russian help might re-form its army and attack again. Certainly the Korean War could have stopped at the 38th parallel, but there was such a huge American army in Korea that it seemed foolish to bring it home before the North Korean regime had been destroyed

and the whole country unified under one anti-communist government. Such were the arguments for continuing the war.

Inevitably, the fighting began again. UN troops invaded North
Korea across the 38th parallel and the casualties came rolling in to
field hospitals and the port of Pusan.

Ruth Stone recalled seeing the corpses arriving too: 'Sometimes
the hospital trains at Pusan disgorged hundreds of white painted
coffins and body bags which we saw loaded onto store ships returning them to the USA.'

Transporting corpses in the height of the steaming hot summer,
was not easy, as Ruth Stone discovered. 'Because of the heat, precious
ice had to be placed over the bodies every two hours. When the
*Maine* docked in Japan the bodies were disembarked first, each one
covered by a flag of its country whilst a military band reverently
played appropriate music as a last tribute.'

So great was the stream of casualties that nurses had little opportunity for resting once all patients were disembarked. They and the
sick-berth staff stripped and disinfected the beds and made them up
for the next convoy. Only after completing this task could the
medical staff sleep, and often it was for twenty-four hours, recalled
Ruth.

But help was at hand for those hard-pressed nurses of the
QARNNS. Three American hospital ships arrived, *Respose*, *Haven*
and *Consolation*. These were superbly equipped and purpose-built
ships. Consequently the *Maine* could leave the Korean war zone and
take seriously burnt soldiers to hospital in Hong Kong.

Their task was never-ending. On 9 October 1950, the United
Nations launched an offensive across the 38th parallel. MacArthur
hoped to encircle and completely destroy the North Korean army.
What he did not know was that on 14 October the Chinese Peoples
Volunteer Army had crossed the Yalu River into Korea in great
secrecy, and by 24 October they numbered nearly 200,000 – three
times more than MacArthur had estimated. And then they waited,
drawing MacArthur's forces into the extremely harsh and mountainous terrain of the north. And the nearer American troops got to the
Yalu river the greater was the risk of provoking the Chinese government into an all-out war.

The ground favoured the more agile Chinese troops over the road-
bound UN forces and they had surprise on their side. The slaughter
began on 1 November 1950 when, just as darkness was falling, thousands of Chinese hit the 8th US Cavalry Regiment. Wave after wave
of Chinese shrieked in at them to an ear-splitting cacophony from

blaring bugles, screeching whistles and shouting used by Chinese to panic their enemies. In two days of fighting, half the US Cavalry were killed or wounded.

Other encounters laid waste to so many UN troops that MacArthur reluctantly accepted General Walker's decision to retreat to secure positions behind the Chongchon River. But retreat was not without risk, for Chinese MIG aircraft had now entered the conflict. Further encounters with the Chinese strained UN medical evacuation resources to the limit. A never-ending stream of wounded flowed by jeep, helicopter and ambulance into the hospital ships and base hospitals at Kure.

That hospital [recalled David Oates] was built on some form of huge roller system devised by the Japanese to withstand earthquakes. The largest ward was the casualty surgical, but there were other wards, orthopaedic, medical, psychiatric, venereal diseases and outpatients – in all about a 1000 beds. There were two operating theatres each with two operating tables. At times we did 80 operations in a day. The routine was occasionally broken when we provided a gynaecological service for Japanese wives of American servicemen. Frequently we did emergency work at night with casualties collected by the 'Emergency Orderly'. They were seen by the Duty M.O. who determined whether surgery was necessary. A theatre technician slept in a room just off the operating theatre to prepare everything at a moment's notice. I used to sleep on a trolley. Sometimes the emergency was to remove someone's appendix. On these occasions it was always 'surgery against the clock' with one surgeon endeavouring to beat the time of a colleague and, of course, to get back to bed as soon as possible!

Our routine surgical work consisted of shattered bones, traumatic amputations, chest and facial injuries and burns of all degrees to all parts of the body. (It surprised me to see how boots, belts and gaiters afforded protection for burns.) Our work was primarily making good corrective surgery and ongoing skin grafting.

From time to time we received casualties from the 1st Commonwealth Division Battle School at Haramura, near Kure, where they trained with live ammunition. Once, when I visited the hospital mortuary I saw the bodies of two soldiers, a Canadian and an Australian. They'd been preparing explosive charges, using gun cotton. One of the dead had his head embedded in his chest cavity as a result of the explosion.

Patients were evacuated from hospital as soon as possible by ambulance train to Iwakuni. From there they went by air to Britain, usually via Kong Kong.

Despite all the casualties from previous offensives, on 24 November 1950 the arrogant, headstrong MacArthur launched his troops into an offensive to reach the Yalu river, telling them the war would be over in two weeks. Within three days the Eighth Army was in serious trouble. Troops were decimated. Typical was the experience of 10,000 US Marines who attacked on 27 November. Waiting for them were 30,000 Chinese. They killed 700 Marines and wounded a further 3,500. In addition, hundreds were stricken with severe frostbite. The rest of the Eighth Army raced back to the 38th parallel.

Now it was clear that the United Nations would have to forget trying to unify the whole of Korea by military action. And from mid December 1950 onwards the course of the fighting depended upon the need to find an honourable way out of the war – a compromise for both sides.

Thus, on 15 December 1950, the Eighth Army withdrew below the 38th parallel, hoping the Chinese would stop when they reached that line. Washington had realized that General MacArthur would have to be held in check too if outright war with the Chinese was to be avoided.

Then fate intervened. General Walker, almost a broken man knowing that he had lost the confidence of his superiors, was hurriedly visiting units to make awards for bravery. The first of these was to award the Silver Star to his son for bravery in action. He had a full day's schedule ahead. Walker was a notorious speed demon, always goading his driver to go faster. On this December morning a South Korean truck suddenly pulled out in front of the General's jeep. Truck and jeep collided. In the tangled mess of steel, General Walker lay dead.

His replacement was General Ridgway, a distinguished paratroop commander, in whose judgment Washington had confidence. And they could deal more directly with him and less with MacArthur.

The UN troops were then holding the line in the hills just behind the 38th parallel. Heavy rain, sleet and snow had swollen streams and made all approaches to their positions difficult, for supply of rations and ammunition and also for the evacuation of wounded. Fortunately, for several weeks there had been little communist activity, but life for the infantry in those forward positions was awful. Many of them suffered terribly from frostbite.

In both the United States and Britain over Christmas, public interest in the Korean War had waned. Headline news from Korea had given way in British papers to the imminent reduction of the meat ration to eight pence a week. The predicament of the 'poor bloody infantry' was not really newsworthy. Soldiers were still being killed and wounded in attacks and counter-attacks, but there was no noticeable gain in ground being made. Wounded were recovered by gallant stretcher-bearers, brought back to regimental aid posts and stacked in unheated medical tents to await treatment. At 30 degrees below zero, blood froze on the wounds. Reports came of medics who kept plasma under their armpits to keep it fluid and of morphine ampoules being placed in mouths. Frostbite injuries afflicted the wounded and the unwounded. As US Marine surgeon Captain Hering stated: 'The only way you could tell the dead from the living was whether their eyes moved. They were all frozen stiff as boards.'[8]

Despite the pressure of work in hospitals receiving casualties, there was still a little time for nurses to relax and socialize. Relationships between the sexes developed easily and naturally into firm friendships and then often into serious romance and marriage. And these were mostly marriages based on commitment rather than temporary excitement. This matches the recollection of Mildred Mitchell, a former QA:

I've heard people say that the very nature of a nurse's work intensified emotions and a tremendous feeling of comradeship developed that supported us when dressing young men with appalling injuries each day. You got to rely on people you worked with and they became an important part of your life. Liking someone easily became more like loving.

The hospital at Kure was not immune to the arrows of Eros. David Oates remembers the romance of QA Sister Burns. She went on to marry the Australian officer in question and invited the whole unit to the wedding reception.

On 7 March 1951, General Ridgway launched operation Ripper and occupied Seoul on 15 March. Now the Korean situation was back to where it was before the invasion from the North. Truman was eager to end the war, there and then. MacArthur was not. He threatened to force China to its knees if they did not withdraw all troops from Korea and allow its unification.

Truman wrote in his memoirs: 'General MacArthur was ready to risk general war, I was not.' He decided to replace him with a more level-headed commander, and he was going to make sure it was done firmly. 'The son of a bitch isn't going to resign on me. I want him *fired*.'[9]

In mid April the Eighth Army advanced slowly forward into North Korea, where the Communists had built up a force of 700,000 men ready to attack the United Nations. On 22 April they struck against the British 29th Brigade front; 10,000 of them slammed into four British infantry battalions. Between half and two-thirds of these 'infantrymen' were national servicemen, some of whom had received only six weeks' training.

> I'd been called up [said Terry Coates], done some weapon training and drill on the barrack square and sent to Japan. I thought it exciting until we suddenly went to Korea, into an absolute nightmare. No one had a clue. We'd been told the first wave of Chinese would attack without rifles, the second wave would have rifles, and so on. In fact most of them had automatic Tommy guns! Then I saw lads near me killed and somehow, my mind still full of training thought, 'Oh we're playing soldiers. These have been killed.' And it's only when things quietened down you realize the truth. They really have been killed. I was lucky and finished up in hospital. In the ambulance a lad next to me said, 'What the hell are we doing here, fighting for a measly four shillings a day?'[10]

The heroism of those four battalions, which lost more than a thousand men in three days of fighting, was described by General MacArthur as 'the most outstanding example of unit bravery in modern warfare'.

The Chinese offensive faded. The line was held. And it became clear to both sides in the conflict that attacks on one range of hills after another was never going to end the war. The time had come for a diplomatic settlement. The American public had lost patience and wanted an end to a war that had already cost them 75,000 casualties.

The Communists too had had enough. Peace talks began in July 1951. But neither side wanted to lose face and appear weak. Consequently, peace talks went on for nearly two years, years that saw some of the most savage and bitter fighting of the whole war.

Nurses could not understand why it was that so many casualties kept coming into their wards when, supposedly, the generals were negotiating for an armistice. Pusan port had never been busier, with three hospital ships, *Repose*, *Haven* and *Consolation*, each with twenty medical officers and forty-one nursing sisters, constantly ferrying casualties to hospitals in Japan.

Sister Gillian Hall (later McNair) of the QARANC, who flew to the Commonwealth Hospital in Seoul, found there were just four QA nurses and two Australian nurses staffing the small temporary hospital housed in a Korean school. In letters home she wrote:

Our patients were utterly astounded to discover that not only are their beds made up with crisply laundered sheets but that there are also 'real Sisters' here to nurse them. . . . But despite the modern appearances of the hospital there is no running water available so that every drop that is needed has to be carried up in cans. It's amazing though, how quickly one can adapt to a tapless situation.

The Commonwealth hospital in Seoul was, to quote Gillian, a 'stop gap between the Field Hospitals such as the US "MASH" which dealt with the surgical emergencies and the General Hospital in Kure. We have a large turnover with most of our patients returning to the front rested and recovered, which I suppose is the real purpose of our being here.'

The living quarters for those nurses could be described as primitive. Water for the showers came from old petrol cans that released a trickle when a piece of string was pulled. There was no privacy, even for the ladies on the four-seater 'thunderbox', as the four holes in planks forming a box over a pit screened by sacking, was called. Gillian McNair (then Hall) recalled in a letter home then: 'I recently found myself sitting next to Matron. Nice as she really is, it really did put me off.'

We hear the distant gun-fire and bombs and it seems a pity that people at home do not take much interest in what's going on. The Americans are doing a magnificent job here and luckily have facilities for most types of surgery.

The peace treaty talks sound as though they might well be fruitful although the South Koreans themselves don't seem to be keen and are in fact upset about this. We can see from the hospital long processions with banners painted with the words: 'UNIFICATION OR DEATH'.

Even when peace negotiations were going well, the fighting never stopped completely. There were battles for relatively minor outposts, remembered vividly by Korean veterans as Punchbowl, Heartbreak, Bloody Ridges, Pork Chop Hill, and the Hook. All were terribly costly in proportion to ground gained. Absurd though it might now seem, during those peace talks the United Nations suffered a further 63,000 casualties. In two years of endless, exasperating, face-saving sparring, soldiers on both sides endured hillside massacres and civilians suffered from massive US air raids.

Fate then intervened again. In March 1953, the 73-year-old Soviet Union leader, Josef Stalin, died.

Two other factors influenced the end of the war in Korea. In the spring of 1953 the United States developed the hydrogen bomb, and in May 1953 the newly elected US president, Dwight Eisenhower, said that he would be prepared to use the atomic bomb against military targets in Korea if the necessity arose.

Finally, on 23 July 1953, just three years and one month after North Korea launched its invasion of the South, the armistice terms were signed and went into effect. The Korean War was finally over.

The most widely accepted estimates show that about 4 million people were killed or wounded during the war. Altogether 54,246 American soldiers died in that war and a further 103,246 sustained non-mortal wounds. Of the men Britain sent to Korea 687 were killed, 2,498 wounded and 1,102 taken prisoner.

What do the nurses and medical personnel now think of that war? David Oates said:

Looking back on those days it is the comradeship I think about and as the years have gone on I have often thought and wondered how those soldiers who passed through our hands are getting on. The broken bones and scarred tissue will have healed, but what of the emotional trauma that these young men suffered?

Half a century later, Korea is still divided into two states at the 38th parallel, but as this closing chapter is being written the presidents of North and South Korea have shaken hands and some families separated for more than fifty years have embraced each other again.

# Epilogue

After the Korean war the British armed services were engaged in a wide range of military operations in a disordered and uneasy world. They helped to contain guerrilla insurrections in Malaya and Cyprus, contributed to international peacekeeping efforts in Sinai and the Lebanon, served in Egypt, East and West Africa, operated in the more conventional war fighting roles in the Falklands and the Gulf, and participated in the intractable conflicts of the Balkans.

With these services, dedicated doctors and nurses showed themselves equal to the task of being ready to share all the risks of active service. The whole story of how far those risks became increasingly fearsome has yet to be officially recognized and made public. But whatever those risks were, one can be sure that the medical personnel involved will be able to look back on their service with the same sense of achievement and justifiable feelings of pride as those youthful heroes and heroines who came back largely unheralded and unsung from wars and conflicts in the hundred years from the Crimea to Korea.

Truly, in words written by Brigadier R.B. Price for the Royal Army Medical Corps hymn:

> Unarmed they bore an equal burden
> Shared each adventure undismayed.

# Appendix

## One Hundred Years of War and Military Campaigns

Crimean War, 1854–1856
Persian War, 1856–1857
Indian Mutiny, 1857–1859
Taranaki Maori War, 1860–1861
Third China War, 1860
T'ai P'ing Rebellion, 1851–1864
Waikato–Hauhau Maori War, 1863–1866
Umbeyla Expedition, North West Frontier, India, 1863
Shimonoseki Expedition, 1864
Bhutan War, 1864–1865
Canada, 1866
The Gambia, 1866
Andaman Islands Expedition, 1867
Abyssinia Expedition, 1867–1868
Lushai Expedition, India, 1872
First Ashanti Expedition, 1873–1874
Malaya, 1875–1876
Baluchistan, 1877
Ninth Kaffir War, 1877–1878
Second Afghan War, 1878–1880
Zulu War, 1879
Basuto War, 1879–1882
Second Naga Hills Expedition, 1879–1880
First Boer War, 1880–1881
Occupation of Egypt, 1882
Sudan, 1881–1885
Karen-Ni Expedition, Burma, 1888–1889

Chin Field Force, 1889
Manipur Expedition, India, 1891
Hunza-Naga Campaign, India, 1891
The Gambia, 1892
Kachin Hills Expedition, Burma, 1892–1893
North West Frontier, India, 1895
Matabele Rebellion, Rhodesia, 1896
Mashona Rebellion, Rhodesia, 1896–1897
Malakand Frontier War, India, 1897–1898
Mohmand Campaign, India, 1897–1898
Tirah Campaign, India, 1897–1898
Sudan Campaign, 1896–1900
Crete, 1898
Second Boer War, 1899–1902
Third Ashanti Expedition, 1900–1901
Boxer Rising, China, 1900
Second Somaliland Expedition, 1902
Kano–Sokoto Expedition, Nigeria, 1903
Third Somaliland Expedition, 1902–1903
Fourth Somaliland Expedition, 1903–1905
Armed Mission to Tibet, 1903–1904
First World War, 1914–1919
Wazaristan Campaign, India, 1919–1921
Arab Revolt, Mesopotamia, 1920
Mohmand Campaign, India, 1935
Second World War, 1939–1945
Korean War, 1950–1953

# References

## 1  Send Them Some Nurses!

1  Cecil Woodham-Smith, *Florence Nightingale*. Constable, 1950.
2  Letter from Queen Victoria to King Leopold cited in E. Longford, *Victoria RI*. Pan Books, 1964.
3  Ian Hay, *One Hundred Years of Army Nursing*. Cassell, 1953. (See also PRO File WO/222/178.)
4  *The Times*, 9 and 12 October 1854.

## 2  Into the Mouth of Hell

1  N. Cantlic, *A History of the Army Medical Department*. Churchill Livingstone, 1974.
2  Anne Summers, *Angels and Citizens*. Routledge & Kegan Paul, 1988.
3  Cecil Woodham-Smith, *Florence Nightingale*. Constable, 1950.
4  Parliamentary Papers, 'Report upon the State of Hospitals of the British Army in the Crimea and Scutari 1854', XXXIII.
5  Cecil Woodham-Smith, *Florence Nightingale*. Constable, 1950.
6  Joseph Lister demonstrated his use of carbolic acid spray to destroy germs in Glasgow Royal Infirmary in 1865. The development of antiseptics after the original carbolic acid meant that operations were no longer a death sentence.

## 3  Order out of Chaos

1  Anne Summers, *Angels and Citizens*. Routledge & Kegan Paul, 1988.
2  *The Lancet*, 9 May 1868, part 1.
3  Anne Summers, *Angels and Citizens*. Routledge & Kegan Paul, 1988.
4  *Nursing Record*, 13 October 1900.

## 4  Nurses Respond to Disasters

1  Medical officer, signing himself 'H.C.' in letter to *Nursing Record*, 13 January 1900.

2  Matron of No. 1 General Hospital, Wynberg, in a letter to *Nursing Record*, 11 December 1899.
3  Letter to *Nursing Record*, 20 January 1899.
4  Anne Summers, *Angels and Citizens*. Routledge & Kegan Paul, 1988.
5  *Nursing Record*, 20 January 1900.
6  Subaltern's letter to *Hospital World*, 27 January 1900.
7  *Nursing Record*, 27 January 1900.
8  Thomas Pakenham, *The Boer War*. Weidenfeld & Nicolson, 1979.
9  Nurse, signing herself 'M.B.' in letter to *Nursing Record*, 16 June 1900.
10  *Nursing Record*, May 1900.
11  Thomas Pakenham, *The Boer War*. Weidenfeld & Nicolson, 1979.
12  *Nursing Record*, 2 June 1900.
13  Thomas Pakenham, *The Boer War*. Weidenfeld & Nicolson, 1979.
14  Ibid.
15  *The Times*, 10 and 11 August 1900.
16  Proceedings of court of inquiry into complaints against men of the Army Hospital Corps employed in the war in South Africa. War Office, 9 June 1882, pp. 1–4 and 8–11.
17  PRO File, CAB 17/12 Keogh to Roberts, 17 January 1905.
18  *Nursing Record*, 11 June 1891. (See also PRO File WO 145/1, Register of Awards for the Royal Red Cross.)
19  H.A.L. Fisher, *A History of Europe*. Edward Arnold, 1936.

## 5  The Challenge

1  *The Poems of Wilfred Owen*. Chatto & Windus 1931.
2  In 1999 Prime Minister Blair's government refused to grant pardons to 306, amongst them six boys, shot for cowardice. Today, former servicemen and civilians claim a pension for what is called Post Traumatic Stress Disorder.
3  Memoirs of Sister Mayne, WW1 Nurses' Memoirs, Department of Documents, Imperial War Museum, ref 82/26/1.
4  Accounts of Misses A. and R. McGuire, WW1 Nurses' Memoirs, Department of Documents, Imperial War Museum. (See also A.J.P. Taylor, *English History 1914–1945*. Clarendon Press, 1965.)
5  The Bible, Numbers 22:22, in which an angel of the Lord stood in the way of Balaam's ass.
6  Lyn MacDonald, *Roses of No-Man's Land*. Michael Joseph, 1980.
7  Diaries of sister M.B. Peterkin, WW1 Nurses' Memoirs, Department of Documents, Imperial War Museum.
8  Notes of Elsie Grey, WW1 Nurses' Memoirs, Department of Documents, Imperial War Museum.

## 6 Usually Quiet on the Western Front

1  As told to the writer.
2  Ian Hay, *One Hundred Years of Army Nursing*. Cassell, 1953.
3  Memoirs of Sarah Huggett, WW1 Nurses' Memoirs, Department of Documents, Imperial War Museum.
4  Hugh Popham, *F.A.N.Y.* Leo Cooper, 1984.
5  Eric Taylor, *Front-line Nurse*. Robert Hale, 1997. (See also PRO File WO/177.1340.)
6  Charles Huxtable, *From the Somme to Singapore*. Costello, 1931.
7  Notes and diaries of Sister Mayne, WW1 Nurses' Memoirs, Department of Documents, Imperial War Museum.
8  Memoirs of Sister Peterkin, WW1 Nurses' Memoirs, Department of Documents, Imperial War Museum.

## 7 A Problem for Nurses

1  Ian Hay, *One Hundred Years of Army Nursing*. Cassell, 1953.
2  Diary of Sister Luard, WW1 Nurses' Memoirs, Department of Documents, Imperial War Museum.
3  Diary of Mayne, WW1 Nurses' Memoirs, Department of Documents, Imperial War Museum.
4  Diary of Elsie Grey, WW1 Nurses' Memoirs, Department of Documents, Imperial War Museum.
5  Diary of Sister Peterkin, WW1 Nurses' Memoirs, Department of Documents, Imperial War Museum.
6  Wilfred Owen, *The Poems of Wilfred Owen*. Chatto & Windus, 1931.
7  BBC interview, October 1999.
8  Siegfried Sassoon, *Memoirs of an Infantry Officer*. Faber, 1918.
9  Wendy Holden, *Shell Shock*. Channel 4 Books, Macmillan, 1998.
10  PRO File WO 177/1734.
11  Wendy Holden, *Shell Shock*. Channel 4 Books, Macmillan, 1998.
12  John Rea Laister in BBC Interview, October 1999.
13  Wilfred Owen, *The Poems of Wilfred Owen*. Chatto & Windus, 1931. Owen was among the final victims of the First World War and his poetry aimed to strike at the conscience of Britain in regard to the continuance of the war. The words 'Dulce et Decorum Est' are often found engraved on stone war memorials in towns and villages.

## 8 Nursing in the Sideshows

1  Letter to the *British Journal of Nursing*, 10 July 1915.
2  Lyn MacDonald, *Roses of No-Man's Land*. Michael Joseph, 1980.

3 Memoirs of Sister Margaret Melrose, WW1 Nurses' Memoirs, Department of Documents, Imperial War Museum.
4 Doris Dickson's letters to the *British Journal of Nursing*, 2 September 1916.
5 Memoirs of Albina Pinninger, WW1 Nurses' Memoirs, Department of Documents, Imperial War Museum.
6 Ian Hay, *One Hundred Years of Army Nursing*. Cassell, 1953.
7 Memoirs of Sister D. Hay, WW1 Nurses' Memoirs, Department of Documents, Imperial War Museum.

## 9 Prickly Heat and Pestilence

1 Letter from the assistant director of medical services to the *The Lancet*, 21 November 1915.
2 Editorial in *Nursing Record*, 20 August 1916.
3 As told to the writer.
4 Ian Hay, *One Hundred Years of Army Nursing*. Cassell, 1953.

## 10 Carnage Incomparable

1 Alistair Horne, *The Price of Glory*. Macmillan, 1962.
2 Letter to the *Nursing Record* and *Hospital World*, March 1916.
3 Charles Huxtable, *From the Somme to Singapore*. Costello, 1990.
4 Ibid.
5 Letter to *British Journal of Nursing*, June 1914.
6 Letter to *British Journal of Nursing*, September 1916.
7 Memoirs of Elsie Grey, WW1 Nurses' Memoirs, Department of Documents, Imperial War Museum. (See also Charles Huxtable, *From Somme to Singapore*. Costello, 1990.)
8 Interview with the writer.
9 Wendy Holden, *Shell Shock*, Channel 4 Books, 1998.
10 Charles Huxtable, *From the Somme to Singapore*. Costello, 1990.
11 BBC interview, 12 October 1990.
12 Ibid.
13 Hugh Popham, *F.A.N.Y.* Leo Cooper, 1984.
14 Memoirs of Elsie Grey, WW1 Nurses' Memoirs, Department of Documents, Imperial War Museum.
15 Memoirs of Sister Essington-Nelson, WW1 Nurses' Memoirs, Department of Documents, Imperial War Museum.

## 11 Year of Decision

1 Letter to the *British Journal of Nursing*, 12 January 1918.

2 Memoirs of Sister Wicker, WW1 Nurses' Memoirs, Department of Documents, Imperial War Museum.
3 Memoirs of Sister Madge Swann, WW1 Nurses' Memoirs, Department of Documents, Imperial War Museum.
4 Hugh Popham, *F.A.N.Y.* Leo Cooper, 1984.
5 Memoirs of Sister Sybil Harry, WW1 Nurses' Memoirs, Department of Documents, Imperial War Museum.
6 Memoirs of Sister Mayne, WW1 Nurses' Memoirs, Department of Documents, Imperial War Museum.
7 Ethel Hutchinson, letter to *British Journal of Nursing*, March 1918.
8 Article in *British Journal of Nursing*, 5 September 1918.

## 12 No Rest for Nurses

1 Marie Stride (ed.), *Celebrating Salisbury Nurses*. Salisbury Nurses League, 1999.
2 Interview with the writer.
3 Marie Stride (ed.), *Celebrating Salisbury Nurses*. Salisbury Nurses League, 1999.
4 Interview with the writer.

## 13 Into Battle Again

1 Cited in Juliet Piggott, *Q.A.R.A.N.C.* Leo Cooper, 1975.
2 Interview with the writer.
3 Alec Adamson's memoirs, given to writer.
4 Juliet Piggott, *Q.A.R.A.N.C.* Leo Cooper, 1975.
5 Penny Starks, *Nurses at War.* Sutton, 2000. (See also Eric Taylor, *Forces Sweethearts*. Robert Hale, 1990.)
6 Alec Adamson's memoirs, given to writer.
7 Interview with the writer.
8 Letter to *British Journal of Nursing*, 20 May 1940.
9 *British Journal of Nursing*, June 1940.
10 Lorna Kite's memoirs, given to writer.
11 *Daily Telegraph*, 26 July 2000.
12 Writer's interview with General Adolf Galland, May 1979.
13 QARANC *Gazette*, vol. 12, no. 1.
14 Martin Allen, *Hidden Agenda*. Macmillan, 1999.
15 Account in *British Journal of Medicine*, March 1941.
16 Personal accounts from nurses of the Coventry and Warwickshire hospital, given to the writer.
17 Ibid.

## 14  Middle East Adventure

1  *British Journal of Nursing*, letter of December 1941.
2  Memoirs of Angela Rigby, WW1 Nurses' Memoirs, Department of Documents, Imperial War Museum.
3  PRO Files WO 170-677 and 272 and WO 177/1245. (See also J.C. Watts, *Surgeon at War*. George Allen & Unwin, 1955.)
4  Memoirs of Angela Rigby, WW1 Nurses' Memoirs, Department of Documents, Imperial War Museum.
5  Pat Hall, in conversation with the writer.
6  *British Journal of Nursing*, letter of 15 January 1942.
7  Alec Adamson's memoirs, given to the writer.
8  Eric Taylor, *Front-Line Nurse*. Robert Hale, 1997. (See also Eric Taylor, *Combat Nurse*. Robert Hale, 1999.)
9  Interview with the writer.
10  Interview with the writer.
11  Poem written by Estelle Lancaster in July 2000 after she had read the experiences of Sister Margaret Jennings at El Alamein in Eric Taylor, *Front-Line Nurse*. Robert Hale, 1997.

## 15  A Damned Close-Run Thing

1  At a gathering of 11th Infantry Brigade in Tunisia attended by the writer. (See also Sir Harry Secombe's autobiography *Arias and Raspberries*. Robson Books, 1989, for an amusing account of this meeting.)
2  PRO File WO/222/178.
3  Cited in Joyce Drury in *We Were There*. Jupiter Press, 1997.
4.  Ibid.
5  J.C. Watts, *Surgeon at War*. Allen & Unwin. (See also PRO File WO/177/1340.
6  Ibid.
7  Interview with the writer.
8  Report in *British Journal of Nursing*, January 1945.
9  Edward D. Churchill, *Surgeon to Soldiers*. Lippincott, 1972. (See also *Royal Hospital Nurses League Review*, Nos ix and x.)
10  Eric Taylor, *Front-Line Nurse*. Robert Hale, 1997. (See also PRO File 177/1340.)
11  Interview with writer.
12  Evidence given at the War Crimes Trial of Lt.-Gen. Ito Takeo, Jan 1948. (See also Winston Churchill, *The Second World War* vol. III. Cassel, 1948. Also Chapter 14 of Eric Taylor, *Front-Line Nurse*. Robert Hale, 1997. Also PRO File WO 235/1107.)

13  See statement by Sister V. Bullwinkel, AGH War Diary, Part 2, 1939–45, 10104178, Australian War Memorial; *QARANC Gazette*, Vol 10, 1994; see also Brenda McBryde, *Quiet Heroines*. Chatto & Windus, 1985; Catherine Kenny, *Captives*. University of Queensland Press, 1986.

## 16  When the Cold War Became Hot

1  Kathleen Harland, *A History of the Queen Alexandra's Royal Naval Nursing Service*. Journal of the Royal Naval Medical Service.

2  Interview with the writer. See also Gillian McNair, *Letters from Seoul* and *British Forces in the Korean War*. Korean Veterans' Association, 1988.

3  Ruth Stone, 'Experiences aboard H.M.H.S. *Maine*', in Ashley-Cunningham-Boothe and Peter Farrar (eds), *British Forces in the Korean War*. Korean Veterans Association, 1988.

4  Trevor Royle (ed.), *War Report: Accounts by war correspondents in Korea*. Mainstream Publishing, 1955. (See also Phillip Knightly, *The First Casualty*. Quartet Books, Andre Deutsch, 1955.)

5  Ibid.

6  Ibid.

7  Ibid.

8  Charles Whiting, *Battleground Korea*, 1998.

9  Richard Whelan, *Drawing the Line*, Little Brown, 1984.

10  Interview with the writer.

# Index